FIT
TO BE
MOM

KIM CAMP

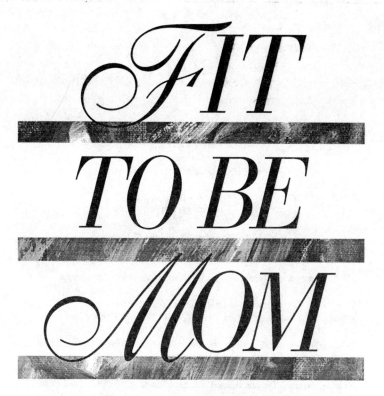

FIT TO BE MOM

Gaining Physical, Emotional,
and Spiritual Balance
in Pregnancy and Motherhood

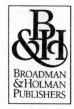

BROADMAN
&HOLMAN
PUBLISHERS

Nashville, Tennessee

4412-01
0-8054-0006-0

Published by Broadman & Holman Publishers
Nashville, Tennessee

Design and Typography by TF Designs, Mt. Juliet, Tennessee

Dewey Decimal Classification: 248.843
Subject Heading: CHRISTIAN LIFE \ WOMEN

Unless otherwise noted, Scripture quotations are from the New American Standard Bible, © the Lockman Foundation, 1960, 1962, 1963, 1968, 1971, 1972, 1973, 1975, 1977; used by permission. Verses marked TLB are from The Living Bible, copyright © Tyndale House Publishers, Wheaton, Ill., 1971, used by permission.

T his book is dedicated to my wonderful husband, Steve, and our precious children, Maxfield, Johnston, Jordan Ruth, Marshall, and Mary Morris. I love you! Thank you for sharing your time, love, and support through the writing of this book. I could not have done this without you!

Most of all, I thank my Lord Jesus Christ who gave the vision for this book and has brought it forth! "I can do all things through Christ who strengthens me" (Phil. 4:13).

CONTENTS

FOREWORD

BY STORMIE OMARTIAN

At the time Kim Camp gave me this book to read and review, she had five children barely six years old and under, the youngest of which was just three weeks old. She looked wonderful, was upbeat and exuberant, and appeared as if she had not been through even one pregnancy, let alone nearly half a dozen. I looked at her in awe and thought, *There is no one more qualified to write a book about staying fit before, during, and after pregnancy than Kim.* That's because Kim's plan of fitness is not just about eating and exercising. It embraces an entire lifestyle that has its roots in fitness of the soul and spirit, as well as the body. She lives the way I do, and that's how I know these principles work for everyone. I only wish I had learned them at an early age as she did, because I would have saved myself a lot of misery.

Kim is a woman of great energy and zest who has her priorities in order and lives what she believes. She is honest and transparent as she shares her personal experiences and inspires us all to be more diligent. Her insights are biblically-based, which puts everything in proper perspective. I've found that one of the best ways to learn how to live is to glean from the sound advice of a person whose own life is a success in all areas. I don't know of anyone else who could have five babies in six years and still look and feel as great as Kim does. She must be doing something right, and the rest of us would be wise to find out what that is.

ACKNOWLEDGMENTS

I also want to thank the following women who have been used by God to mold me into the woman He wants me to be. You have impacted and continue to impact my life.

Marietta Maxfield—my mother, my friend, and my faithful prayer warrior, who encourages and challenges me in every chapter of my life. A gifted attorney and author, her editing skills have taken this book from my computer to the publisher.

Doris Morris—my grandmother and my mentor, who asks the tough questions and leads me to the Scriptures for the answers. At eighty, she is the most totally fit woman that I know, for her beauty both inside and out is more evident every day.

Meredith Maxfield Christensen—my sister and friend whose energy and enthusiasm inspires me to see the higher path where the Lord has called me.

Ruth Camp—my mother-in-law and exhorter who keeps me focused on what really matters in life.

Stormie Omartian—Her inspiration, encouragement, and faithfulness to stay totally fit as a wife and mother are invaluable.

Kim Boyce Koreiba—who has shown me that priorities can be kept when outside demands are high and that it's worth it not to compromise!

Debbie Smith—one of my few friends who started having multiple children before Steve and me. Her faithfulness as a wife of a traveling husband and mother of five has blessed me. She and Michael have opened their home to families who need accountability, prayer, and fellowship in the midst of our everchanging culture.

Kathy Thomas—her gift of laughter, her practical, and committed style of mothering three small boys and friendship have made a lasting impact on my life.

Cile Scanlan—her great smile and incredible mastering of many talents from nursing to decorating to event planning have shown me the need for balance as a wife and mother.

Karthi Masters—my dearest friend through many stages in life who now mothers her first baby boy.

Tiffany Wilmont LeBlue—my new friend and choreographer so essential to this project. She is incredibly brilliant and wisely balances mothering her precious daughter with using her God-given talents.

Halle Searcy—her gentle and quiet spirit coupled with her fervent excitement about being a first-time mom has been amazing and inspiring.

Carol Frazier—a wonderful mother of three who lives the totally fit life. She is living proof that a woman can get back in shape after pregnancy, and she inspires me not to give up even if it takes a year!

Nan Cox—with three kids three and under, her fun approach to mothering has encouraged me to be more practical and nurturing.

Kathy Harrell—a great mother of five, with her youngest the same age as my oldest and her oldest soon in college. Kathy helps guide me in my role as a mother.

Kathy Peel—this most creative mother and best-selling author has shared the trials and triumphs of parenting with humor balanced by a godly foundation. She has taught me the value of being a family manager.

Sara Olsen—her four children are within days or months of four of ours. The Lord has used Sara in my life as "iron sharpens iron" to help keep me focused on His Word.

Doreena Williamson—a partner with her husband in ministry, she has inspired me about being a helpmate to my husband and keeping my priorities balanced with ministry and motherhood.

Mary Trapnell—my dear friend whose two boys are one month younger than our two girls. She is faithful to pray for our family and this project and holds me accountable to "walk my talk."

Stephanie Coker—after successfully raising three beautiful daughters, she has mentored our young mothers group in loving commitment.

Tara Wilson—a part of our family since moving to Nashville, she has a heart for missions. Her research has helped shape the moral fitness part of this book.

Cindy Tripp—who has worked miracles with the book after it was delivered to the publisher. She's been Johnston's Sunday school teacher and a new friend.

Nancy Norris—Thank you for teaching me how to thread the theme throughout the book and encouraging me to share the story behind the facts.

INTRODUCTION

BY STEVE CAMP

I n the world of late night television (one of my favorite times of the day) we are literally bombarded by what has become known as infomercials. Of all the late night ads, exercise is one of the most popular. Over-tanned physiques ripple with superior muscular definition at every circuitous turn; the hardest of exercises are performed with such ease that we wonder, *Do they really get to look this good from just twenty minutes a day three times a week in the comfort of their own homes?*

From home gyms to thighmasters, ab crunchers to treadmills, mountain bikes to healthriders, from buns of steel to dancing, sweating, eating, and cruising to the oldies with Richard—the infomercials have made their mark and are here to stay. But if you're like most couch potatoes (this spud included), you need to hear the clearcut clarion call to better health and a more active, energetic, robust life. You need nothing more than the encouraging words from a loving, caring spouse bellowing with the intensity of "I can't believe the Browns are really leaving Cleveland" saying *just do it!*

1

But seriously, shooting straight from both of my hips, the secret to having great health, like anything else in life, is finding and maintaining *balance*. That is the key! To grow physically, socially, emotionally, and spiritually requires balance in living. Extremes in exercise can cause muscle damage, fractured bones, dislocated joints, etc. Extremes in our everyday living will produce similar results: damaged relationships, fractured friendships, and dislocated marriages. Therefore, the right amalgam of discipline, devotion, and diet; encouragement, exercise, and edibles; caring, calisthenics, and cuisine is not only advantageous but crucial to obtain the quality of life you want.

That's what makes *Lifersize* so refreshing and valuable. This program doesn't call us to diets, fads, or quick-fix-it ideas that for the most part are inimical and antithetical to every day living. What it does do is to *call* us— or rather *confront* us—to examine ourselves, to take an honest look at our habits, values, and priorities with razor-sharp clarity. Then it equips us with some tools to order our days with lifestyle choices that will positively impact the way we live. *Lifersize* is not Peter-Pan pat answers. It was not invented in a lab or by the latest professionals on maternity recovery or "conceived" in an exercise facility with those whose metabolism has been in warp drive ever since birth. *Lifersize* was born from living in the pots and pans of everyday life by a housewife remembering some well-given wisdom from a father to a daughter—my wife! It is real solutions, regardless of age, regardless of environment, regardless of circumstances or economic standing, to equip us for the challenges that we all face twenty-four hours a day, seven days a week. *Lifersize* is simply conforming one's day to patterns to have the quality of choices based on faith, family, and friendships.

I am a firm adherent to the axiom, "What we believe determines how we behave." The voices that we listen to shape and mold our values, character, and morals. As a Christian, the voice that compels and conforms me is the truth of God's Word—the Bible.

You might be thinking what could the Bible possibly say about health, fitness, and physical exercise? The pages of Scripture are not silent. "For bodily exercise profits a little, but godliness is profitable for all things, having promise of the life that now is and of that which is to come" (1 Tim. 4:8, KJV).

Do you see the balance? Training and exercise are profitable, but we must keep them in balance with that which is to come. Godliness, our time spent in devotion to the Lord, should be the first thoughts on our minds and the premier desire of our hearts—before we commence with the workout schedule and daily tasks of the day.

I am honored to have been asked by my wife Kim to write this introduction. I am proud to be called her husband. She is an exceptionally disciplined woman, a gifted mom, and a faithful wife. She is my best friend—and that means we share the trials as well as the triumphs! As parents of five children ranging in ages from six to six months (three boys and two girls), we both know the need and the struggle to not become a slave to the urgent but to constantly remember what's really important. I believe this is what makes *Lifersize* so beneficial—it focuses in on what is truly important!

In writing this I know I am sealing my own fate. I'll have to finally lose my own love handles—the ones I have come to admire these past many years. Traveling 200,000 miles a year I thought would give me the excuse not to *just do it!* Through this program Kim not only takes away my excuses but she replaces them with viable, clear, positive alternatives. This is a program for life, one that you can tailor for *your* lifestyle and family needs. It deals with the whole person. We both trust this will encourage you not only to maintain healthy choices for a more sound and vigorous life, but will also uplift and provoke your faith to mature and grow in the grace and knowledge of our Lord Jesus Christ.

So get ready for a great adventure with Kim and the *Lifersize* team! Not many of us will do extraordinary things in our lives. But if we do the ordinary things of living faithfully, we can make an extraordinary contribution to our family, friends, church, community, and ourselves!

So remember, begin each day with the Lord and time in His Word, keep family a priority, nudge your husband to join you in this program, enjoy your kids, throw away the scales, stop counting calories, don't let anyone catch you reading too many labels in grocery store aisles, and once in a while eat dessert first—for life is too short!

THE FOUNDATION

"Your father's plane has crashed and there are no survivors." The memory of those words still ring in my head as I reflect on the man who so powerfully impacted my life that what he instilled in me continues to affect the whole direction of my life. Those were the hardest words that I have ever heard, yet the Lord used the tragedy of losing an extraordinary father who lived eighty years in forty to start my journey. At age seventeen I began to discover not just who I am, but most of all, who I am in Christ and what is the foundation upon which to build my life.

Throughout these pages, I will share the total fitness principles which my father laid out for me at the age of twelve and special ways in which my parents, grandparents, and precious others have shaped and influenced my life. My prayer for you is that you will incorporate the *Lifersize* perspective to effectively change or enhance your daily habits and improve every aspect of your life. As you launch your own total fitness program, you will discover that total fitness is broken down into three areas:

1) physical fitness 2) moral fitness, and 3) spiritual fitness.

PHYSICAL FITNESS

Our culture has been obsessed for half a century with how we look: fashion design, make-up, and a flab-free body. Standing in the grocery store line for the fiftieth time that month and surprisingly finding myself without any children (besides the precious little one inside my tummy), I took those many moments to read all the magazine covers and skim through a couple of articles. It was amazing to see that every cover, regardless of which type of magazine it claimed to be, had at least one "flash" about getting in shape quick, headlined "Six Weeks to a Bikini Body" or "Lose 20 lbs. in One Week." Obviously, this approach appeals to over 70 percent of the American people who are overweight or to the 85 percent who think that they need to get really skinny to look great. It's not a new revelation that our culture is obsessed with skinny bodies, and most people are desperate for a quick result.

What is new is the current focus on staying healthy. As we learn the benefits of a healthy lifestyle and as we impart these *Lifersize* principles to the next generation, the diet and exercise rollercoaster can come to an end. Our children too will benefit.

Being physically fit means more than looking good on the outside; it means feeling physically fit through healthy eating and exercise habits. Our physical appearance reflects the fitness of our bodies, as well as our daily interaction with our family, friends, and business associates. Although no one formula works for everyone, certain guidelines light the path to "total fitness."

MORAL FITNESS

In every area of life, whether big or small, I am impacted by a variety of integrity-testers. Once as I was working on a total fitness article for a Christian magazine, I took off on a twenty-four-hour trip with a schedule of to-do's that should have been stretched over ten days. As I raced to turn in my rental car with only thirty minutes until my airplane departure time, I made a conscious decision to skip the gas refill. I marked the fuel level box "half full," and I handed my rental contract to the employee, a good-looking young man about twenty-five years of age. He scanned the contract and then commented, "I'll mark your gas box full on the contract because the company will charge you a fortune to fill it up." As I turned down his offer, he looked at me as if I were really foolish, but what I heard him say sounded like, "Good for you!"

And the story continues. My flight landed, and after I had shuttled to my car, I paid the parking lot attendant, who handed me a bill as change, which I pocketed without looking at it. The next morning I noticed a ten-dollar bill had been handed to me by mistake, instead of a one-dollar bill. I quickly called to advise the company that a nine-dollar error had been made in my favor. The supervisor was so thrilled with my honesty that he insisted that I keep the nine dollars, which was more than enough to compensate for the higher gas charge for the rental car!

Tears filled my eyes as I was reminded of God's hand guiding every detail of my life. I call it *grace* whenever God covers my mistakes, when He even makes an impossible schedule possible. Whether or not I am repaid for small points of integrity, and regardless of the risk involved to state the truth, I have determined that it is well worth it to do what is right. I know that only God's grace makes my integrity possible, so I am forever grateful. I am reminded in Psalm 50:14–15: "What I want from you is your true thanks; I want your promises fulfilled. I want you to trust me in your times of trouble, so I can rescue you, and you can give Me Glory!" (TLB)

As a mother, I find it so challenging yet vital to show godly, moral behavior in all of my words and actions before my children. Knowing that they watch and listen holds me accountable—and the times that I fail to make the right decision, I humbly ask forgiveness and pray for God's grace to cover mistakes that I played out before their eyes.

So what is moral behavior? What about the times that right and wrong don't seem so clear cut? Webster defines *moral* as "conforming to a standard of right behavior." This leads to our final fitness area, spiritual fitness. God's Word is the standard by which we live. Having a vibrant spiritual foundation is what builds that moral fiber within us so that we can make the right decisions in life. At times the Bible is not clear on a particular issue, and we must seek the Lord and allow Him to show us the right answer.

SPIRITUAL FITNESS

The way we live our lives reflects the foundation upon which our life is built. Will it crumble under pressure or withstand the test of trying times? My junior high years were vital formative years in my life. I was blessed to have a youth pastor, Bob Alexander, who ingrained in us 1 Timothy 4:12: "Let no one look down on your youthfulness, but rather in speech, conduct, love, faith and purity, show yourself an example of those who believe." Bob did not offer "entertainment only at cheaper rates" to pass the time while our parents were studying the Bible. I will never forget the Sunday that he gave a powerful call to the youth.

Bob said, "If you know that you're a Christian and you are not spending daily time in God's Word and in prayer, being discipled and discipling, and sharing Christ with your friends, then you are not walking in the will of the Lord!" Wow! Were we really supposed to do all of that at twelve years of age? He laid out a plan to read through the Bible in one year; on Monday nights at a Bible study (which included youth from twelve to eighteen, which was *really cool)*, we could ask any question about the Word or about life and discover the answers from God's Word.

At the same time my father started me on a healthy, physical fitness plan; and then through my Mom's faithful prayers and example, I was drawn to Jesus' call to build my life on the solid foundation of a covenant relationship with our Lord Jesus Christ. My mom realized that her prayers had been answered when she found me three nights in a row, wide awake, way past my bedtime, reading the Book of Revelation. It's incredible to look back and see God's hand moving steadily with every year in ways far more effective and much greater than I could imagine or dream.

In Paul's epistle to Timothy, the Lord challenges us to "Continue in the things you have learned and become convinced of, knowing from whom you have learned them" (2 Tim. 3:14).

One of the greatest gifts that my parents gave to me is the ability to learn from others. "The way of a fool is right in his own eyes, but a wise man is he who listens to counsel" (Prov. 12:15). They taught me to love and appreciate constructive criticism because it stretches and challenges me to examine my position and determine whether a change needs to be made. While I do not assess the validity of what I believe or say or even my own strategy by another's feedback, I find constructive criticism does influence the outcome.

One of my weaknesses is being opinionated. Just as Maria said in *The Sound of Music,* "I am far too outspoken; it's one of my greatest faults." I have learned that I can get beyond my own opinion and grow to value the viewpoint of another; then I can evaluate their input and possibly change my opinion. Through considering another's viewpoint, I allow myself to examine several positions and studies, but I constrain myself to a conclusion consonant with God's Word.

This principle is found in two of my favorite passages: "Do nothing from selfishness or empty conceit, but with humility [this is the key] of mind, let each of you regard one another as more important than yourself; do not merely look out for your own personal interests, but also for the interest of others" (Phil. 2:3–4,) and from the Book of Proverbs, "Without consultation, plans are frustrated, but with many counselors, they succeed!" (Prov. 15:22). Humility is the key which is necessary for us to seek wise counsel.

Now that I'm married to a wonderful man and we have five children, the Lord has placed an urgency in my heart to share these principles with you because I can say, "They work!" My hope is that you will commit to incorporate the *Lifersize* principles into your everyday life and determine to *never, never* quit. I encourage you to live a balanced life, one which is physically, morally, and spiritually rooted and grounded in the firm foundation of a vibrant relationship with the Lord Jesus Christ!

PART I

PHYSICAL FITNESS

WHAT IS YOUR MOTIVATION BUTTON?

For a teenager, fatherly advice is a mighty motivator, but "who likes whom" or "crushes" can change the course of your life. I was having a "date with Dad" at McDonald's on the Plaza in Kansas City, Missouri. As I devoured my favorite meal—a Big Mac, large Coke, fries, and a box of animal crackers—my dad shared with me the importance of healthy eating and exercise habits.

The plan that Dad described would definitely eliminate everything that I was eating. He said, "Kim, if you'll drink water, juice, and milk instead of soft drinks and eat three balanced meals a day, you'll be a whole lot healthier." Dad then cushioned his proposal for monumental change with motivating details. "In fact, Kim, the chances are that you'll never have to diet—if you cut out the excess salt, fried foods, and snacks. Also, if you'll do ten or fifteen minutes of exercise every day and something aerobic three to five times a week, you'll never have to worry about being out of shape."

Visions of my favorite meals danced in my mind's eye, and I knew that Dad's way of life would involve quite a

13

sacrifice. Dad could tell what I was thinking, so he added, "Kim, if you'll start this now, you'll be so thankful when you're twenty, because all this will be a habit." I knew he was right, but at twelve, it didn't seem that important. Anyway, I thought worrying about being in shape was something you do when you're old or married. So I dismissed it—until the next afternoon.

Unknown to me, my dad made his point by using peer pressure of the most powerful kind! The next morning my junior high crush, Bruce Brackeen, poked me in the stomach and said that I was getting a "pooch." Well, that did it! There was *my* motivation button! I couldn't believe that Bruce Brackeen noticed or even cared. All of a sudden, that little plan Dad had discussed with me the day before became very important.

I immediately started on Dad's program; and now, almost twenty years later, a Big Mac and fries is not the least bit tempting. While I know that this anecdote is especially motivating to those who are teenagers or have teenage daughters, the unanswered question remains, "How does *Lifersize* translate for women aged twenty, thirty, forty, or older when unhealthy habits are already established?"

POWERFUL MOTIVATORS

All of us are motivated differently. Listed below are some factors that may spur you to establish healthy habits. In fact, I hope that one or more will magnetize with your motivation button(s) and pull you into *Lifersize* for a lifetime.

- Energize your body and and feel 100 percent better with consistent exercise and a healthy diet.
- Revitalize your organs through exercise by causing oxygen to flow through your body. Don't use feeling tired as an excuse to skip exercise because exercise will give you a second wind and add two hours of clear

thinking at the end of your day! After lunch, a twenty-minute power nap can do wonders for the "midday blahs." It stretches your productive hours and prolongs your patience and gentleness with your children.

- Guard against heart disease by keeping your weight consistent with a lifetime commitment to *Lifersize*. Steady weight control will add years to your life and be a valuable gift to everyone who loves you.

- Maintain a high metabolic rate. Once you reach your best weight, then you can keep your size without constantly counting calories. Your metabolism will speed up and stabilize without your being a slave to a particular diet.

- Eliminate constipation. Along with a steady metabolism comes consistent bowel movements. Consequently, you probably won't have to deal with hemorrhoids (unless you're pregnant, but we'll talk about that soon).

- Stay the same size, and stop worrying about fitting into *those* pants this week! They will always fit (unless, of course, you're pregnant!).

- Be content with your size because you are on a healthy eating and exercise plan. Realize that the Lord has made everyone unique! Can you imagine that the human body came from the dust of the earth? You are a miracle of God's creation, and you can praise Him for His miracle. Your success depends on not comparing yourself to anyone else!

- Relieve stress naturally with physical activity. For busy moms like us, this is a must!

- Be an example to your children to make physical fitness a priority. Realize that it will be hard to teach your kids something that you don't do yourself.

- Save money you might spend for a "tummy tuck" by keeping your abdominals in shape through crunches and aerobic exercise.
- Look healthier and younger!
- Participate in your favorite sports because you're in shape. *Lifersize* will increase your "wind," reduce puffing and panting after five flights of stairs, tone your muscles, and reduce your chances of injury from a fall caused by flabby muscles.
- Prevent injuries by consistently keeping your muscles toned. Consult your doctor before embarking on any new exercise plan if you have had an injury requiring rehabilitation (such as a knee or back injury). Conform your exercise to your doctor's guidelines.
- Break the smoking habit. Dr. Ken Cooper, who was a good friend of my father's and now a leading expert in exercise and health, says, "Consistent exercise will help keep your heart and lungs healthy, and it is the most effective way to break the smoking habit or to keep it from even starting!"
- Guard against eating disorders with steady *Lifersize* principles for lifetime health management.
- Guard against osteoporosis, which decreases bone strength and causes fragility.

MOTIVATORS FOR EXERCISE DURING PREGNANCY

Here are some special motivators for pregnant or soon-to-be pregnant moms:

- Ensure a healthy pregnancy and a speedy recovery by using the *Lifersize* program to get into shape before your pregnancy. During pregnancy, use a modified program and increase your chances for a safe delivery and a speedy recovery.
- Help prevent swelling in the wrist and ankles.

- Keep the abdominal muscles strong to support the back during pregnancy and for labor and delivery.
- Use leg and calf exercise to decrease leg cramps.
- Guard against constipation at a time when most women take extra iron, which causes constipation. Hemorrhoids are common during pregnancy and immediately thereafter, and exercise is a recommended preventative, although no guarantee against the problem.
- Get extra oxygen to your baby and yourself, too!
- Help prevent varicose veins and guard against those tell-tale stretch marks.
- Build your self-esteem with healthy and toned arms and legs during pregnancy when your body is growing and changing.
- Get back in shape more easily after the delivery by practicing healthy habits. You're also more apt to let the weight come off naturally, too.
- Have the strength to take care of your baby and keep up with your other children as well!

SUCCESS BREEDS SUCCESS

These are a few reasons to incorporate a healthy eating and exercise program into your daily routine! Since success breeds success, I want to share a story that may become a key motivator for you from my wonderful friend Beth.

> My son Austin and Kim's oldest child Maxfield met on the first day of preschool and became best friends. It's amazing how the Lord develops incredible friendships for moms through the friendships of their kids. Like Steve, my husband also travels a lot, so Kim and I would spend time together on the weekends. One night, I asked Kim how she got back in shape after having a baby. Her youngest was about six months and mine was two, yet even though other people complimented me on my appearance, I knew that my body was still not back in

shape. I was starting to get really frustrated. So Kim told me about the exercise program that her dad put her on when she was twelve, and then Kim challenged me to make exercise a part of my daily routine and to do something aerobic three to five times a week. I was at such a point of frustration that I was willing to try anything.

After about a month, I was wearing shorts, and both my cousin and my husband (who had been out of town for three weeks) commented, "Beth, your hips and legs look better then ever! What have you been doing?" Well, that made it all worth it. It really was working! I want to encourage you that it's never too late to get in shape—and getting on a healthy and consistent eating and exercise program that becomes a part of your life really works! I spent two years vacillating between gimmicks for diet and exercise and giving up. With *Lifersize*, I have a program that works and a friend to hold me accountable!

Having babies and wanting to look good for our husbands (or at twelve, your junior high crush!) are two great motivators for having a healthy body. Sometimes my friends and I will laugh and say that God made men to keep women in shape, but as we get older it seems that several of the other motivators intensify. It is hard to develop a habit once we become set in our ways, but experts say that it takes only thirty days to establish a habit.

My grandfather made a drastic lifestyle change at age thirty-nine. Unfortunately, it was not by choice. Grandaddy was a trial attorney until he suffered a massive heart attack and was in recovery for one year. He moved from a fast-paced lifestyle to a small room on the first floor of his home. He was told to take it easy and do only minimal exercise for the rest of his life. The doctors gave him five to ten years to live if he slowed down and six months if he returned to his previous lifestyle.

Well, my grandfather is an amazing man. He discovered new research that exercise and weight control, as well as a specialized diet, might reduce the risk of heart disease. He started swimming, then walking, and jogging regularly. The more he exercised and carefully monitored his food intake, the stronger and better he felt. His routine consisted of regular exercise (tennis and hand ball twice a week, a daily fast walk), a thirty-minute midday nap, a daily dose of lecithin and vitamin E, and no saturated fat in his diet.

These guidelines along with healthy eating habits have brought great reward. Right before Grandaddy's eightieth birthday, he experienced some chest pains. The doctors thought that the pains were probably caused by his heart, but the tests could not find anything wrong. In fact, this eighty-year-old man, who had suffered a massive heart attack before age forty, now has the arteries of a sixteen-year-old! Since his brush with death forty years earlier, he has been the "king of preventative medicine," taking precautions with his health at every turn. Using the data from forty years ago and the present, the doctors plan to use Grandaddy Carloss as an example that diet and exercise drastically reduce the risk of heart disease! What an inspiration! (And the pains have not returned!)

So find what will motivate you. Write it down and post it around your house. Then, call a friend to hold you accountable and invite her to join you in the program. In just *one month* you will definitely see the difference!

chapter three

EAT RIGHT;
DON'T EVER DIET

F reedom from dieting was a powerful motivator for me to exercise and to eat right. As Dad explained to me years ago, dieting without exercise is ineffective because exercise tunes the metabolism. We must burn about 3,500 calories to lose *one* pound, and exercise speeds up our metabolism. If we exercise without modifying our diet, then we will become frustrated with turtle-slow results. Balanced eating habits coupled with exercise will eliminate the drudgery of dieting and the health hazards of anorexia (starvation) or bulimia (overeating followed by self-induced regurgitation) which is so prevalent among women from middle school age and into adulthood.

SEVEN GUIDELINES
FOR HEALTHY EATING HABITS

1. *Eat three balanced meals a day.* Cutting back on your caloric intake and fat is vital to the process of losing weight. Remember, too, that while your body requires no more than ten grams of fat daily, it does require a small amount of fat. Balance is the key in what you eat—and

when. The expression, "breakfast like a king, lunch like a prince, and dinner like a pauper," must have sprouted from the experience of our ancestors. Eating close to bedtime overtaxes the digestive organs during sleep when the body needs to rest. Food unburned by exercise turns into unburnable energy, better known as fat.

Since 1980, the definition of a balanced meal has changed. Food advertisements used to emphasize the importance of a meal centered around a meat, such as rib-eye steak or fried chicken, with heaping portions of the "four basic food groups." Today, we know to avoid cholesterol-building foods with high fat content such as gravies and sauces and fried foods.

I've listed below a few of my favorite healthy choices for each meal. You can combine them in a way that best fits your appetite and time schedule.

Choices for Breakfast:
- two low cholesterol eggs lightly seasoned with fat free-cheese (and busy moms should know microwave eggs taste really good and kids like them too!)
- medium-sized bowl of fresh fruit
- one to two pieces of wheat toast (add honey or low-fat preserves if you are in a maintenance program)
- juice or milk (skim or 1/2 percent)
- decaffeinated tea or coffee
- bowl of fat-free granola or some other type of high-nutrient, low-fat cereal, with fresh fruit on top
- whole wheat waffles or pancakes with light syrup

Choices for Lunch:
- salad with a healthy, light or low-fat dressing
- turkey sandwich on whole wheat bread (watch the condiments, choosing the light or fat-free mayonnaise dressing)
- fat-free yogurt with fresh fruit or granola

- grilled chicken sandwich, turkey burger, or garden burger
- healthy leftovers from the night before (as a mom, I have learned to like and to value these "quickies.")
- steamed veggie plate with a baked potato (choose toppings wisely depending on your goals)
- sherbert or frozen yogurt with fresh berries

Choices for Dinner:

(Many of the lunch choices can also be eaten as a full meal in the evening.)

- grilled chicken, seafood, lean meat, or wild game
- more fresh veggies
- fresh salad with grilled chicken or beef
- homemade veggie pizza with a light tomato sauce on a whole wheat crust
- sorbet or any kind of fat-free, light dessert (like angel food cake—my favorite!)
- fresh berries with a light whipped topping

Salads are important, but watch the dressings you use! My friend uses lemon juice on her salad instead of dressing, an effective way to lose weight. Once a desired weight is attained, you can maintain it by switching from lemon juice to healthy low-fat dressings. Eating out at restaurants can also be healthy, especially in today's health-conscious environment. Ask the chef to prepare steamed veggies without the addition of any oils. You can also split a meal with your spouse or date at a restaurant. At our house Sunday brunch out is followed by "cereal night." The kids love it, and it certainly makes Sunday night more restful.

Remember the importance of decreasing your food intake as the day progresses and eating small portions of balanced meals. At the same time, it is important to eat until you are satisfied so that you will not be tempted to snack.

Recent studies show that the best way to lose and maintain your weight may be to eat six small meals rather than three full meals daily. This supports another nineties "buzz phrase," food is fuel! Skipping meals actually slows down the metabolism; eating the right foods along with consistent exercise speeds up the metabolism. My friend Kamee has found that this system best controls her weight. But be careful: If you choose the six-meal system, make sure that your food intake does not increase.

The nutrients your body requires are found in natural fruits and vegetables (five servings daily) supplemented by trace minerals and fish and chicken several times per week.

2. *Avoid snacking on junk foods.* Snacking on chips, sweets, or anything handy is not the way to curb the appetite between meals. Instead, if hunger gnaws at your stomach between meals, reach for a piece of fruit or eat an entire bowl of grapes or a sack of carrots (when I am pregnant, I crave the grape/carrot snack). Watermelon, celery, or broccoli are all great choices for snack foods. You'll want to cut these up when you come in from the store so that they are ready when the hunger pangs strike.

Smoothies are fun, healthy, and easy to make. Put two cups of frozen fruit and two fresh bananas in a blender, fill to the brim with juice (orange or cranberry or mixed), blend, and *voila*, a smoothie! Another favorite smoothie recipe is to combine one pint of frozen strawberries (no sugar added); one-third cup juice plus Lite powder (full of nutrients from fresh fruits and vegetables), and mix with cranberry juice in the blender.

3. *Eat desserts in moderation.* If you have a "sweet tooth" (like I do), then it's important not to deprive yourself of all desserts. My friend Kathy could eat dessert with every meal without gaining weight. Another friend, also

named Cathy, feels that she gains ten pounds everytime she looks at a dessert. Once again, balance is the key! If you're trying to lose weight, limit dessert to one day per week or to special occasions. Whenever you order a dessert, make sure it is fabudelicious and split it with a friend. Try to order fat-free or low-fat yogurt or some kind of sherbert or sorbet. If you're a chocolate lover, then try fat-free hot fudge on raspberry sorbet—it's just as incredible as calorie-galore chocolate cake with raspberries! Once you reach your desired weight, you can enjoy dessert from time to time. Guard against the return of bad habits, however.

Here's a quick note on cellulite: This fatty deposit under the skin, which looks like cottage cheese, is one of the greatest battles for women, so if you have it—you're not alone! I didn't struggle until I started having children, and now it creeps onto my thighs and bottom during pregnancy and then takes months to go away, but *it does go away*! If you have always struggled with cellulite, it will take a while. Be encouraged, though; if you stick to a healthy eating and exercise plan, you will see results!! Do extra repetitions on problem areas with the *Lifersize* isolated exercises. Cut back on fatty foods, but don't eliminate all fat from your diet, since your body needs some daily fat intake. It's too easy to give up and say, "Oh, this is just how I am" or to become obsessed with the fact that it's there. If you are patient and faithful to healthy habits, it will disappear naturally and not come back! (Unless you're pregnant again, of course!) But the joy of a child will far outweigh the frustrating process of smoothing out the "cottage cheese."

If you are built like Kathy with a "K," then you should eat dessert in moderation for nutritional reasons. You should watch your sugar intake and be aware that up to twenty teaspoons of sugar are in just one piece of cake. If you're built like Cathy with a "C," these lifetime guidelines will work to keep your body trim. You should cater to your sweet tooth only on birthdays and Sundays—and then cut those desserts in half when you do indulge.

4. *Stay away from fried foods!* Some people (like my husband) crave fried foods more than they crave desserts. If fried foods are not your special love, then it is definitely best for your health to entirely banish them from your diet. If you love a big plate of french fries or onion rings, apply the law of moderation as with desserts. My friend Stephanie loves fried chicken and says that it seems un-American not to eat fried chicken at least once a week. After much discussion, we hit on a compromise. Her family first cut back to twice a month, then only once a month. This satisfies their craving yet diminishes the health hazard of excessive fried foods.

5. *Drink gallons of water, milk, and juices!* In other words, stay away from soft drinks. As my dad always said, "Water is the best drink in the house." Drinking eight glasses of water per day is the best advice I know.

Also, stay away from caffeine! I know that this is diffi-cult for coffee drinkers, but thankfully, there is decaf! (And if you are not already a coffee drinker, don't start!) I didn't realize how much caffeine affects the body until I became pregnant with our first child. At the time, I drank iced tea as if it were water because it was the only drink available when I was away from home other than soft drinks. When I found out about the harmful effects—that caffeine eats the vitamin B in the body like Pac Man—I went off "cold turkey." After a month I felt better, and now if I drink something with caffeine, I get head-aches and feel dizzy. (Plus, my Grandmother Dearie has always told me that vitamin B_6 is a "cure-all" for sickness during pregnancy.)

My friend JoAnna lived with us for fourteen months after our third child, Jordan Ruth, was born, and she was addicted to her favorite soft drink. (Notice that "addicted" is in the past tense.) I know that some are reading this and saying, "There is *no way* that I could give up my favorite soft drink!" However, one year later JoAnna got concerned about her health, and she started exercising and eating right—and she gave up soft drinks. She will tell you that it wasn't easy, but it has been well worth it! Several years ago my mom decided to add exercise to her daily routine and to drop coffee from her daily liquid intake. She was successful for three years—until the two hours she had allocated for daily exercise began to diminish; and then the exercise became sporadic. To continue her busy work schedule, she allowed coffee to creep in. Today, she is making a quality commitment to *Lifersize* principles: working exercise into her daily routine, cutting coffee to one daily cup, and "sharing" desserts on special occasions.

6. *Don't add salt or sugar to food on your plate.* Of course, if you're following a recipe, you will add salt and sugar as directed, but refrain from adding sugar to a drink or salt to your meal once it is served.

7. *Always eat before 8 P.M.!* Did you realize that your body must complete the digestion process before you go to bed? If you eat too late, your organs are working instead of resting the first two hours of sleep. Eating close to bedtime also causes the body to store the unburned calories as fat. If you get really hungry before bedtime—or if you're an athlete who's played a night game—then eat fruit or drink a big glass of milk before going to bed.

FIVE HEALTHY TIPS FOR PREGNANCY

With four of my pregnancies; I experienced the normal nausea and occasional vomiting, but with my fourth baby, Marshall, I was *so* sick that I experienced occasions when I could not take care of my three children (ages three and under) at a time when my husband was traveling constantly. During this time the Lord provided through the "angels" of His selection. One evening I was in the den lying on the couch and feeding Jordan Ruth in her high chair. Maxfield and Johnston were at the kids table on top of the splat mat. I was praying that the smell of food would not cause me to make another trip to the toilet. I walked to the kitchen to get applesauce, and the next thing I knew, I was startled by the doorbell and realized that I had fainted. I was lying on the floor with applesauce smattered all over the den carpet. The kids were screaming and wondering what had happened to their mommy. I had fainted before, but it was always quick and I could get up and go on. This time, however, I must have been lying there for about ten minutes, and the Lord had sent a friend to my aid.

I answered the door, and Wendy handed me a bowl she had borrowed. I tried to act normal because her children were waiting in the car, and she seemed to be in a hurry. However, she quickly assessed the situation and graciously offered to help. She brought her children inside, fed mine, and helped me clean up. She even helped get my children in bed.

How grateful I was that God knew my need before I even asked and that He does not allow us to be tested beyond that which we are able. Wendy was clear evidence of God's perfect and timely provision!

Here are some healthy tips I've used during pregnancy.

1. *Eat balanced meals—adjusted as necessary!* During the first and last trimesters of your pregnancy, you need to split up your breakfast and dinner since most women feel nauseous during the first trimester and experience heartburn during the last trimester. Eating five or six light meals throughout the day buffers these common pregnancy problems. However, if you experience the kind of

sickness that I had with Marshall, then eat *whatever* your body will digest! The only foods that I could keep down then were hamburgers and plain baked potatoes, so I put the guidelines on the shelf. (That was a big diet change for me, since I normally eat four to five hamburgers a year.)

When you are in your middle trimester, regular balanced meals seem to work for most people. You can also enjoy fruit and smoothies between meals.

2. *Eat desserts in moderation.* During pregnancy, my metabolism *stops*, and I gain about forty to fifty pounds. I have found that if I cut back on sweets and increase my aerobic exercise from three to five times per week to five to seven times per week, my muscles will remain toned and my weight will continue at a healthy balance.

A quick note on weight gain: As long as you eat right and exercise, don't concentrate on your weight. The priority is the baby growing on the inside, not the outside appearance. Some people gain twenty pounds, and others gain fifty pounds or more. Allow your body to gain what it needs. This is not the time to diet if you considered yourself ten pounds heavier than your target weight at the time you became pregnant! One way to judge whether you are gaining unnecessary weight is to measure your thighs when you find out you are pregnant and once a month thereafter. Your legs should stay within an inch of their original size during pregnancy. If they exceed one inch in gain from the beginning of pregnancy, evaluate your food intake to see if you need to cut back on desserts or fatty sauces. If these are not a regular part of your daily meals and you are exercising regularly, then know that your body needs to gain a little more.

During my first pregnancy, I learned that there is a lot of caffeine in chocolate (which is absolutely my favorite dessert of all time) so I eliminated chocolate from my diet—even to the point of not eating the tiny chocolate squares given as a pseudo dessert on airplanes. Then when I was pregnant with my second child, I read research that there wasn't a lot of caffeine in chocolate, so I decided to eat it in moderation. Of course, moderation to me was a large piece of chocolate malt cake (with dinner, of course). I learned that this was definitely a caffeine overdose for a six-month baby in the womb! Little Johnston did the chocolate dance to the caffeine tune until about 2 A.M.— and I discovered that a little chocolate square on the airplane is chocolate in moderation!

3. *Drink lots of water.* When you're pregnant, drinking lots of water deserves a super emphasis! My friend Carol, who is an expert on nutrition, told me that it's not just drinking lots of fluid, but getting the proper amount of water every day to prevent dehydration. She emphasized that iced tea and even healthy juices do not count in your minimum eight to ten glasses of water a day. I buy small bottles of fresh water and put them in the refrigerator so I can grab one to take with me everytime I leave the house— which is eight to ten times a day with five children.

When I'm in my nauseous stage of pregnancy, however, I do alter my no-soft-drink rule and take a carbonated drink to calm my stomach. At other times you couldn't pay me to have a carbonated drink, but when I'm feeling sick it tastes as good as water!

I know that we hear a lot about water retention during pregnancy. Even though you may think that drinking a lot of fluids cause swelling, this is not true! When you exercise regularly and replace fat with muscle, the muscle will store the water and keep your body hydrated, especially during pregnancy. Then you will naturally release the fluids and maintain a healthy balance.

4. *Eliminate salt.* Salt contributes to temporary problems during pregnancy. This is definitely a good time to start eliminating excess salt from your diet.

5. *Eat before 8 P.M.* This is an important health guideline during pregnancy, especially if you're experiencing

heartburn. Also, during pregnancy our bodies store extra fat, and the later in the day we eat, the fewer calories we burn. Any calories retained is fat gained! My friend Mary usually stays up until 11 or 12 at night, but when she's pregnant, bedtime is no later than 9 P.M. If you go to bed earlier, try to eat by 6 P.M. so that your body will have at least two hours to properly digest your dinner.

Now, an added note to the nauseous: Sometimes it helps to have something on your stomach before bedtime. If this is your problem, drink a glass of warm milk, have a piece of bread or some crackers, and put something by the bed to eat as soon as you wake up.

At the time of this writing our fifth baby is one week old, and I'm quickly remembering how ravenous a mother gets when nursing. I feel as if I can't get enough food. During the first four to six weeks after delivery, you should ease back into a regular eating and exercise program. If you're "starving" because you feel as soon as you "inhale" your food, the baby "sucks" it all out, eat healthy snacks and extended meals even though you're probably craving something else (chocolate!).

I hope that these guidelines that I've learned from both experience and the wise advice of others will help you to have a more relaxing and restful pregnancy, recovery, and beyond. Remember that every baby is unique just as every one of us is unique, so there isn't a "down pat" answer for having a successful diet and fitness program or a stress-free pregnancy and recovery. To end on a very positive note, I just talked with a young lady who is three months pregnant with her second baby and both pregnancies have been nausea-free. She doesn't know her secret, but she's thankful and living proof that it could happen (to you!). Take these principles and apply them to your life when applicable. Ask the Lord for strength as you start to establish healthy habits that last a lifetime!

EXERCISE IS
A WAY OF LIFE

ow many times have you been asked about your most embarrassing moment? I have at least one hundred times and could give one hundred different stories. Moments of embarrassment seem to follow me as a puppy follows its master, but I guess that's one thing that makes life so much fun. Although I can think of several which occurred during the last month, one of my most embarrassing moments occurred when I was sixteen years old at a week-long camp. I was with ten other young girls I did not know very well in a cabin with one counselor. We were having fun figuring out which one of us was going to fall in love with which cute guy and if this "growing experience" at camp was really worth it. Well, I didn't think anything about my little exercise program; it was just part of my daily morning and evening routine. I honestly didn't notice that others weren't doing it.

Imagine my shock when my cabin peers imitated me doing my exercises in a very exaggerated and funny skit in front of the whole camp! I wanted to just disappear, but I had to laugh and admit (even to my newfound crush) that I did this every day. Six of the girls from our cabin either came to the Lord or started growing in the Lord that week, and we continued to be dearest friends throughout high school and college. They still give me a hard time, but in college people were well aware of my daily routine, and some even made it a habit of their own.

This routine was a part of me. If people were interested and asked, I would share it with them, but I was not aware that *Lifersize* would work for everyone. Because I started daily exercise at twelve years of age, I had never experienced the frustration of gaining and trying to lose weight. Then I became pregnant and gained around forty pounds with each baby. This program was so ingrained in me that I just kept on doing what I was doing. After I had each baby, I was afraid to try some kind of temporary diet because I had seen so many of my friends lose weight and then regain it within several months.

After my fourth baby, I realized that this program really works for me even when my body is overweight. I began to realize that the program could work for other people who also struggled with their weight. Everyone seemed to "get back to normal" at a different pace, but within twelve months everyone who had a healthy eating and exercise program during pregnancy—and continued with the same basic lifestyle after the baby—didn't have to ride on the diet and exercise roller coaster that becomes a way of life for so many women. This realization coupled with a lot of prayer and leading from the Lord compelled me to want to share these principles with other women.

THE BASIC EXERCISE ROUTINE

My basic routine consists of isometric and kinetic exercises. This means that the muscle is isolated when you exercise; you can concentrate on working that particular muscle rather than doing the movement. (You may also choose to use light handweights [two to five pounds] for muscle resistance and toning three times a week.) Regular weight-bearing exercises build strength and endurance and guard against bone loss and the debilitating effects of osteoporosis later in life.

The goal is to replace fat with muscle. An important point to remember is that muscle weighs two and one half times more than fat, so you can't be concerned about your weight! Instead you should focus on how your clothes fit. You may only lose a few pounds, but go from a size 10 to a size 8. After having a baby, I monitor my progress with a tape measurer. By checking my inches, I know how far I have to go until I am back to my normal size.

This basic routine covers every part of the body. It may sound like a lot, but as you get used to it in your daily life, it is quick and easy, yet *very effective!*

If you're in the pregnancy/recovery stage of life, a few guidelines should be followed. Depending on which trimester you're in, you can vary the same basic exercise. Remember that a pregnant woman should not lie on her back for more than one minute at a time after her fourth to fifth month of pregnancy. Especially when you work your abdominal muscles, perform the exercises standing, sitting, or on your side. Also, if you have not been previously working out with weights but would like to start, wait until about six weeks after you've given birth.

Side Stretches. Lift your arms to the sky and reach for 12 counts. Now place one arm on your hip, knees slightly bent, feet shoulder width apart and facing forward, lift one arm up and then stretch it to the side. Hold for 12 counts. Don't bounce; hold steady. Repeat for the other side and hold for another 12 counts.

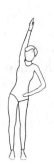

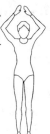

Pull downs. Both arms up, now bend at your elbows pulling down behind your neck for 12 counts. Make sure that you keep your neck in line with your spine. Concentrate on using your back and shoulder muscles. (This is great for that "bra strap overhang"!)

Shoulder rolls: Drop your arms to the side for 8 shoulder rolls. Lift shoulders up and back. Push those shoulder blades together. If your neck and shoulders ever feel tense during the workout, stop and do some shoulder rolls.

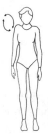

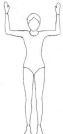

Butterfly. Hold your arms straight out to the side, bend at elbows, and count 12 butterflies. Pull your elbows together and back out. As your arms go back, really work your back and shoulder muscles and as they come forward, use your pectoral/chest muscles. Now bring your arms together above your head, then elbows out, and now elbows together and out for 12 upper butterflies. (This gives definition to your upper back.)

Bicep curl. Put your arms down by your side for 12 bicep curls. Bring arms up at the elbow and down. Really concentrate on working your muscle rather than just moving your arms up and down. (This builds stronger arms for carrying the baby.)

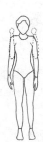

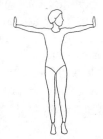

Wallpush. Place your arms out to the side with hands flexed to work the triceps. Look at your hand and pretend to push against a wall. Hold for 12 counts; repeat for the other side.

Tricep extension. This continues to work the triceps, ensuring that you won't get those flabby arms when you're fifty! It also begins to work out the lower body. Face sideways with your feet staggered. Place the arm opposite your front leg along the line of your leg. Bend your elbow up and 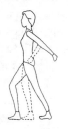 back. Now extend your lower arm. Concentrate on working your tricep and also bend and straighten your leg along with your arm. Do 12 with each arm.

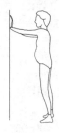

Kinetic pushups. This final upper body exercise is an isolated way to do push ups especially when you are pregnant. (If you're in your first trimester, you may do push-ups ladies style. If you're in your final trimester, you may want to do your push ups standing against the wall.) Place your arms straight in front of you with hands flexed and bend your elbows moving forward and back, forward and back for 12 counts. Concentrate on working your pectoral and arm muscles as if you were actually doing pushups. (This works the entire upper body and is a quick substitute for ladies-style pushups.)

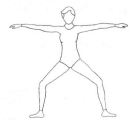

Pliès. Place your feet a little farther than shoulder width apart. This exercise may also be performed while doing most of your upper body exercises. This gives a little extra workout for the legs. Make sure your knees are directly over your toes with your knees facing the same direction as your feet or you could eventually cause harm to your knees. Bend your knees and glide back up. When you come up, squeeze your buttocks and your abdominals together. Pull yourself up with those muscles. Glide up and back down for 12 pliès.

Kegals. Continue doing your pliès and add some kegals. A kegal is the tightening and release of the pelvic floor. It strengthens the muscles in the pelvic floor and helps you to push that baby out! Also keeping those muscles strong will greatly assist in the recovery. Bend your knees and stay down. Place your hands on your knees, tighten your abdominals and keep your hips tucked under. Now tighten the pelvic floor and release. (This same muscle is used to stop the flow of urine.) Tighten and release for 12 kegals. This exercise can also be done at stop lights or any time that you're sitting or standing still during the day. You'll really appreciate these later (and your husband will too!).

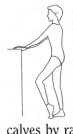

Calf raises. Place arms straight out in front of you for balance, unless you feel more stable with your arms out to the side. If you still feel unbalanced, hold onto a chair or a sturdy piece of furniture. Feet shoulder width apart and facing forward, knees slightly bent. Keep your upper body stationary and work your calves by raising up to the balls of your feet and rolling back down. Raise and hold, now roll down. Continue for 12 calf raises.

Leg lifts.

- *Back leg lifts*—When preg- 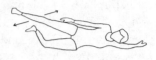 nant, lie down on your right side, using a support- ive pillow under your head if needed. Bend your bottom leg and flex your top foot. Take your leg back and in, back and in for 12 lifts to work your hamstring. Concentrate on using your muscle to lift your leg. Feel that muscle work. Then point your toe to work your buttocks for 12 lifts back and in. When you're not pregnant, you may lie on your stomach.

- *Outer leg lifts*—Place your 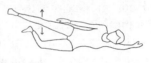 upper leg directly in line with your body, flex your foot, and lift your leg, up and back, up and back, for 12 lifts. Then with toe pointed for 12 lifts to work your outer thigh. Concentrate on your abductor muscle.

- *Inner leg lifts*— Straighten your bottom leg 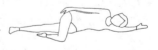 and place top leg in front of you with knee bent com- fortably to work your inner thigh. Flex your foot and move your leg up and down for 12 lifts. Keep it in line with your body and really work your abductor muscle. Then point your toe for 12 lifts. Next slightly lift leg and make small movements back and in for 12 lifts. Then walk yourself up slowly and turn to work the other leg.

Crunches. If you are *not* preg- 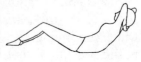 nant or if you are in your first trimester *only*, lie on your back with knees bent. If you need extra support, place your hands gently behind your neck. Make sure that you lift with your stomach muscles and not with your hands or shoulders. Place your hands gently behind your neck and lift forward and back, forward and back. Your head should be in line with your spine as if you have an orange under your chin. Start with twelve to twenty-five crunches in the morning and again at night. Then work up to fifty in the morning and fifty in the evening.

If you are in your second or third trimester of pregnancy, lie on your left side and bend your knees slightly. Then crunch your stomach muscles while on your side. You may prefer to do your crunches while sitting or standing. This will prepare your stomach muscles for labor and keep them well worked so that once the baby comes, your stomach will nestle back in place—that is, as long as you are continuing a healthy eating and exercising program! Strong abdominals support the back and remove the uncomfortable pressure from your back especially during pregnancy.

I know this seems like a lot to remember, but once it's a part of your everyday life for just thirty days, it will become second nature.

PUTTING IT INTO PRACTICE

Now for some creative ways that can help you put exercise into your daily routine.

Start your *side stretches* the minute that you roll out of bed. It feels invigorating to reach up and stretch out your upper body. Then as you walk to the bathroom, continue with your *pull downs, butterfly,* and *bicep curls.* Start your *pliès* in the bathroom as you finish your *bicep curls*—then . . . "go to the bathroom"[smile]. Go to the sink and do the *wallpush* and the *tricep extension*— while continuing to work your legs. I usually do my pushups at night, but if you have time, do the *kinetic pushups* standing up. Now do your *calf raises* while brushing your teeth. Then wash your face and continue with the *pliès* and some *kegals*. Next, turn on the shower and while it's getting hot, do twenty-five to fifty *controlled crunches*. Take a shower. While you're putting on your make-up and/or fixing your hair, do your *leg exercises* standing up—the side (the abductor muscle), center (the abductor muscle), and back (to work the hamstring) on each leg. Each exercise should be done for eight to sixteen counts depending on the amount of time that you have in the morning.

In the evening, I do the same basic routine while getting ready for bed except for two changes. I do my crunches while I dental floss my teeth, and then (when I'm not pregnant), I roll over and do my ladies-style pushups. When I'm pregnant, I sit up and do the *kinetic pushups*. Three to five times per week during the news on television, I exercise with light handweights (which takes about five to ten minutes) followed by something aerobic for the other twenty to twenty-five minutes of the news program.

When you're in the first four to six weeks of recovery, continue doing the basic exercises, but do fewer repetitions at first and work back up to your normal routine. Slowly working back up to aerobic exercise is important too. Since I have just had our fifth baby, I am quickly reminded of how uncomfortable it is to do anything more than moderate walking if you're nursing. That's because it takes a little while for the breasts to regulate the amount of milk the baby actually needs. Of course, before leaving the hospital, ask your doctor when you can begin exercising. My doctor encourages women to begin these basic exercises, or Target Training, immediately if things went well in delivery. (This will vary if you've had a C-section or many stitches due to a radical episiotomy.) I did not do *any* exercise until one month after delivery with our first child, Maxfield (I had many stitches and an infection), and with our fourth, Marshall (it was a tough delivery and surgery).

Consistency is the most important point to remember. The number of repetitions of a particular exercise is not as important as exercising everyday; it is imperative that you do not skip doing your exercises. One concentrated and controlled movement is much more effective than ten fast uncontrolled movements. Performing six to eight repetitions of an exercise in a steady, controlled manner brings more results than sixteen to eighteen repetitions done at a fast, jerky speed.

An example of this routine is given in the *Lifersize* videos. These videos will help you to get acquainted with the proper way to do these exercises, which can be done quickly with the Target Training section on the video. Then incorporate the routine into your everyday life and use the complete video tape for your aerobic exercise. I know that if these areas are not currently in your life, it may seem impossible to add *one more thing* to your routine. Once these exercises become your own habit, however, you will be surprised at how little time it does take to reap a lifetime of benefit. I guarantee that every minute spent is *well worth it!*

ACCENT
THE NATURAL

I have always admired Grace Kelley, not only because of her natural beauty and acting ability, but also because she maintained a realistic, balanced perspective while being "Princess Grace." Though she lost her life suddenly in her prime years, Grace Kelley is forever intriguing. As an economic advisor and author, my dad had the opportunity to develop many wonderful and interesting friendships. One evening he sat next to Grace Kelley at a dinner party and related the challenges of having two "almost teenage" daughters. He mentioned his special concern that my sister Meredith and I thought we were almost eighteen, especially in the way we dressed and our insistence on wearing makeup. Princess Grace's response was unforgettable, "My 'rule of thumb' is that a girl can never go wrong if she accents the natural beauty God has given her!"

Well, this was definitely something Dad passed on to his daughters! My motivator button had been punched! I started to notice the girls that I thought were really pretty and not just the ones that looked "older." I was drawn to the girls who enhanced their natural features

43

through make-up rather than allowing makeup to domi-
nate their face. Soon the blue and purple eyeshadows,
thick black mascara, and prominently outlined bright
lips were replaced with natural eyeshadows, occasional
light mascara, and a natural lipgloss.

My dad also helped me to appreciate the natural way
God made me in the areas that I had tried so hard to
change. I was born with thick, curly hair; every girl that I
admired had beautiful "normal" straight hair. For two
years, I had ironed my hair and used thinning scissors as
my solution to having beautiful (and acceptable) hair.
Also, most of my friends had gorgeous, bright blue eyes.
Mine were hazel—which meant that my eyes definitely
weren't blue; on some days they were green and other
days they were kind of brown or somewhere in between.
Since one of Dad's entrepreneurial ventures was Morgan
Optics, a contact lens manufacturing company, I found
that I could get contacts (even though I didn't even wear
or need glasses) that would make my eyes blue! Well, that
year my song was, "All I want for Christmas is Big Blue
Contacts . . ."

BEING THANKFUL FOR HOW WE LOOK

Trying to change these two basically unchangeable
parts of my appearance began after Vacation Bible School
when I was eight years old. My mom had taught about
the wonderful missionary Amy Carmichael whom I have
since come to greatly admire. As a little girl with big
brown eyes, Amy had prayed to the Lord for blue eyes as
bright as the ocean. In VBS, Mom only told a little of the
story each day, so I went home the first day thinking that
if Amy could pray this, so could I—and I could also pray
for straight hair! I prayed very diligently that night for
straight hair and blue eyes and went to bed with full con-
fidence that I would wake up with my prayer answered.
At 6 A.M., I ran to the mirror expecting to see a change,

but there I was, looking the same way that I did the night before. I was so disappointed with the answer to my prayer. I did remember that when I was five I had prayed for Mr. Jones at church who had cancer and the doctors had given him three months to live. Now three years later, he was still alive and doing well. If God had answered yes to such a big prayer, how could he say no to this little request?

I returned to VBS that day, and Mom finished the story. Amy's eyes hadn't turned blue either, and God had a very good reason! When Amy became an adult, she was called to work in India. To live and minister among the people, she needed to look like them. Although she had brown hair and brown eyes, she had light skin. So she darkened her skin with coffee grains and the Indian people thought that she was one of their own. The Lord used her mightily; she rescued girls from being temple prostitutes and discipled many during her years in India. The Lord knew the purpose for her life long before she was even born and had fashioned her physical appearance to fit her calling in life. How comforting to know that He has a special purpose for our lives and has molded us both inside and out to fulfill His mighty work in us!

Unfortunately, this incredible truth didn't quite sink in for me at the age of eight. However, it did begin to build an attitude of trust in the sovereignty of God. Because of my Christmas request, Dad was very "tuned in" to what I thought was important. He encouraged me to let my hair be naturally curly and he assured me that there were a lot of blond-headed, blue-eyed girls, but that I was extra special to have blond hair and hazel green eyes! So although I was caught up in the excitement of "blue contacts," I was prepared through the story of Amy Carmichael to be thankful for the unique way God made me. I realized that I, like Amy, would someday understand and appreciate God's providence in making me just as I am.

THE NATURAL LOOK

Rather than trying to alter our appearance, we should play up our natural strong points and be thankful for the areas that we can not change. I've tried to make "accenting the natural" my motto even when my face breaks out (which definitely happens in a major way when I first get pregnant, after I have a baby, and when I stop nursing). Even though my eyes look swollen, I've found that it's better to lightly and naturally cover up the blemished areas, than to pile on a whole bunch of make-up and announce to the world that I depend on make-up to look more beautiful. Of course, there are definitely times to dress up and look glamorous; but even then we should enhance, not remake, our natural appearance.

My friend Sara is so beautiful without any make-up; however, she feels "naked" without it. As a child she had short hair and was often mistaken for a boy, so since her early teenage years she has worn a lot of make-up. Her husband constantly tells her how gorgeous she is without make-up, and she's slowly starting to wear less. Men appreciate women who don't spend a lot of time on their appearance. It only takes several minutes to enhance our appearance in a very natural way.

This fresh, natural look begins with good skin care. Find a good product line for your face (it doesn't need to be expensive) and faithfully wash, tone, and moisturize your skin every morning and every night. My mom also taught me to not forget to moisturize my neck, as well. Sleeping on your back (unless you are five to nine months pregnant) will also help prevent premature aging because gravity holds your skin back and in place. You spend at least one-third of your life sleeping, so it really does make a difference.

Former Miss America, Debbie Barnes, spoke at a weekend conference that I attended my seventh-grade year. She made an indelible impression on me concerning how girls should dress. She simply said, "Dress for Jesus." At the time I thought this statement was pretty trite. However, it's been an unconscious guideline for me since that conference. This doesn't mean to wear long dresses and skirts and constantly downplay your figure, but it does mean not to draw attention to the parts of your body that can be distracting and cause men to stumble.

So focus on your physical assets and experiment to see which styles look best on you. Don't feel like you have to wear the latest styles. Wear what looks good on you and feels comfortable. For example, I have never felt comfortable in the wide-legged, extremely loose fitting pants. I've tried to keep my wardrobe up to date with the shoes that I buy and with shirts that have in-style necklines and collars. Many dress shops encourage you to bring in your favorite outfits and the salespeople can update your wardrobe with a few pieces. This is a great way to maximize your dollars and still feel in style!

MATERNITY FASHIONS

When I'm in that three- to six-month stage of pregnancy, I feel like wearing a button that says, "I'm not fat; *I'm pregnant!*" I have the hardest time figuring out what to wear without abandoning myself to big shirts and leggings from the beginning. Through some helpful advice and some experimenting, I've found some tricks to get through the fifth month of pregnancy without wearing maternity clothes.

The first hint is the rubberband trick. Put a rubberband through the buttonhole of your pants, shorts, or skirt and then loop the two ends around the button. As you grow, you need to get bigger rubberbands, but this will usually work through about the fifth month of pregnancy. At first, you can still tuck your shirt in and then blouse it over the rubberband. When you're about four months pregnant, a stretchy or big belt and a jacket will work, and it's very slimming.

Also, my friends who are two sizes bigger than I am normally will lend me their clothes for four months and then again for a few months after I have the baby. This is another great option, especially since they offered to lend me their clothes without my asking. Another idea is to go to some secondhand sales and pick up a few things. This is a really wise option if you're planning on having more children. And, of course, your husband's big rugby and polo shirts work great with leggings or shorts. These few ideas will lessen your time and investment in maternity clothes. Then you can start wearing them when you're showing enough to feel good and can look pregnant in maternity clothes rather than just feeling heavy.

I remember being three months pregnant with my *first* baby and wearing maternity clothes that swallowed me; yet I didn't care, because I wanted everyone to know that I was pregnant. By the time I needed them, I was so tired of those same clothes! With the other pregnancies, I've used these helpful hints and found that I was in maternity clothes just long enough to enjoy them. My friend Kim, who has one adorable little boy, says that during pregnancy she accented the areas that weren't rapidly expanding and then played down the areas that were constantly growing, like the waist/stomach and the hips. This is a good guideline when picking your clothes during pregnancy. Black is always a good color especially when wearing leggings. The "baby doll" dresses that stop right above the knee look really flattering in the final trimester and then they're also nice and comfortable right after the baby is born.

SEEK THE LORD

A final part of accenting the natural goes far beyond our outward appearance. With every baby I find people (usually those I don't know well) love to come up, touch my stomach, and give me all kinds of unsolicited advice. (If I ever come up and do that to you, please just smile and walk away—I'll get the hint!) I hope that you will read a lot on pregnancy and parenting and then seek the Lord to see what is your (as Chuck Swindoll calls it) "natural bent." Proverbs 15:22 says that there is wisdom in many counselors. It's important to gather all the information and advice from those we respect and then go to the Lord and see what He wants for our family.

My friend Sara and I have so much in common, yet we are very different as well. We know that the Lord ordained our friendship because our kids are the exact same age. Our first two boys are two days apart. Her second and my third are two months apart (I had the privilege of seeing her little girl born), and our youngest boys are three days apart. So we have had many conversations about childrearing. We both do a lot of research and seek lots of advice, yet we've come to two different conclusions on the way we handle babies.

I received a wonderful book when Maxfield was three weeks old entitled, *My First Three Hundred Babies* by an English nanny, Gladys West Hendrick. Well, that book told me everything I needed to know! Before I had Maxfield, I had never even changed a diaper! Not only did it explain about bathing and feeding the baby, but it also told me how to put the baby on schedule. The wonderful part about this concept was that at two weeks old Maxfield's 2 A.M. feeding was eliminated and he would sleep from 10:30 to 6:30 in the morning; by eight weeks old he slept 6:30 P.M. to 6:30 A.M. (He still sleeps twelve hours, if he has the opportunity.) This schedule also included regular nap, feeding, and play times. Gladys

Hendrick wrote that scheduled babies are welcomed members of the family who fit into the routine of the home and are given stability through knowing what to expect. Furthermore, it's not what the baby does, it's what you do about it that sets the tone for the baby. We took her basic principles and schedule and made it work for our family. Although I did not agree with everything that she said, I found many good points to consider.

Since then, I have come across another wonderful tool called *Preparation for Parenting* by Gary and Anne Marie Ezzo which balances the *300 Babies* book with biblical principles. The Ezzos material emphasized the importance of parent-controlled scheduling versus child-centered parenting. We have balanced a strict schedule with the importance of using the schedule as a guideline and allowing ourselves to be flexible. We also don't want our parenting to be controlled by the clock. Each child has special needs.

Through the grace of our Lord, our home, even with five kids barely six and under, has a relatively peaceful environment in which the children feel stability. The first six weeks after the baby is born, I just don't get an adequate amount of sleep; I know that I am not as tuned in to the children's needs as when I'm getting enough rest. As the mom of the family, I need to get enough sleep to function. The kids' schedule gives me the ability to know that I can sleep, catch up on my responsibilities, as well as enjoy fun times with my friends, when the children are napping or resting and after bedtime at night. The books also tell how to schedule two or more children as well as twins or triplets. Parent-controlled scheduling has complemented my personality and enabled me to be an effective mom to my five young children.

When my friend Sara's baby was still not sleeping through the night at several months old, I thought that I was doing her a big favor by sharing this information

with her. Well, she had done her own research and felt
that "demand feeding" (i.e. letting the baby naturally find
its own schedule) was the best solution for her little boy.
He did eventually get on his own schedule, and her children are very godly and mature. Now that our boys have
reached the age of six years, I cannot say that there are
any significant characteristics in either of them as a
result of our different parenting styles. However, if I had
used Sara's method with my five children, I would have
been a "basket case"; and she assures me, that if she had
used parent-controlled scheduling with her three children that she would have "gone crazy." Parents must
seek the Lord and His direction regarding the baby
parenting method which is best suited for their family
unit.

As in most areas of life, we also must find balance. We
can't focus so much on what "works for us" that we lose
sight of the clear-cut biblical principles for parenting
that need to be followed and not questioned. However,
when it comes to examples like Sara's and mine, we must
seek the Lord so that He can "accent the natural"
through us!

PART II

MORAL FITNESS

YOU DON'T HAVE TO BE A SIZE 4!

While I was a radio, television, and film major at The University of Texas, one of my classes studied the impact of hard-sell and soft-sell commercials. The bottom line was that commercials appeal to the audience through sexual connotations. Whether subtle or very direct, the message was the same: "This is how you should and can look if you use our product." If you want to be beautiful in other's eyes, you must be extremely thin and tall, with perfect skin, and always look attractive. As a result, many women strive for this "perfect" look—and it is not always possible. Some women are naturally tiny, and with healthy eating and exercise habits, they will be a size 2 or 4. Others can healthily eat and exercise and will always be a size 12 because they are naturally taller and/or larger boned. God made every person unique. Don't set a goal to reach a small size or certain weight. Instead, be the size the Lord made *you*. Healthy eating and exercise habits is the real goal—and one which will have an effect on your size and weight.

It's amazing how two people in the same family can be diametrically different in physical appearance, yet evidently related as indicated through mannerisms or expressions. I'm built like my grandmother on my mom's side, and my sister is like our great-grandmother on my dad's side. Meredith is statuesque and taller than I; when both of us maintain healthy habits, she will still wear a size bigger than I do. She is beautiful and is custom-made for her tall and handsome husband Jon.

UNHEALTHY COMPARISON

Wonderful freedom can be found in godliness with contentment. Contentment is the opposite of unhealthy comparison. No matter how "together" your life may be, you will meet those who seem to be more "together." Only moral fiber grounded in spiritual truth develops satisfaction with yourself and with the circumstances of your life—where God has placed you. Only moral fiber produces the ability to learn from other people and to be genuinely excited about the Lord's blessings in their lives. Comparing ourselves with others can be very dangerous because it produces dissatisfaction, and the unhealthy mental attitude of comparison can actually lead to covetousness. The Bible strongly speaks against coveting: "You shall not covet your neighbor's house; you shall not covet your neighbor's wife (or husband) . . . servants, ox, or his donkey or anything that belongs to your neighbor" (Exod. 20:17). *Covet* means to deeply desire and crave for yourself something belonging to someone else. This is not always a material thing; it may be a physical or spiritual attribute that either intimidates you or creates distance with that other person.

I'm not talking about admiring a quality that another displays. Learning from someone else and growing from their example are wonderful, wise traits to develop. Comparing yourself to another in an ungodly way is focused on obtaining that which belongs to another, whether it is actually a person we know or an image we have fixed in our minds.

After having a baby or when needing to lose a lot of weight, you'll find the weight comes off quickly at the beginning. About six weeks after a healthy program is started, the weight continues to come off consistently but more slowly. At this point the process can be discouraging, and the temptation arises to compare yourself to others and try to get a speedy result. I am at that six-week mark in my postpartum recovery, and I have to pray for patience and not pay attention to the advertised "fast diets." Hang in there. Remember that if you just had a baby, it took nine months to gain the weight. If it's been a while since you had a baby, then you've been carrying the weight even longer—so give yourself about a year and know that when you do reach your natural, desired weight you can remain that size by continuing healthy habits.

A 1994 article in our Nashville newspaper *The Tennessean* entitled "Starving for Perfection" underscored the danger of appearances. The focus was on "a young gymnast who lost her life because she thought she had to reduce to a size 0 in order to attain the 'Perfect 10.'" This young woman, who was twenty-two, died after succumbing to bulimia and anorexia. At the height of her career, she weighed ninety-five pounds. When she died, she weighed only sixty-one pounds. Christy Henrich's death jolted the gymnastics world, but it should be a wake up call for all of us. The article challenged parents: "We cannot afford to let our children believe that they will only be perfect if they lose weight. In fact, we cannot afford to let our children believe they need to be perfect!" This powerful statement is applicable not only to children but also to women from adolescence to adults of all ages.

Anorexia and bulimia are very dangerous diseases with 200,000 new cases each year and a mortality rate of 5 to 15 percent. Eating disorders begin with the unhealthy comparison with others and a resulting dissatisfaction with a person's unchangeable physical facts. Some eating disorders arise when some women have become discouraged with missing their weight goals on the diet and exercise rollercoaster. They then try to take a shortcut to achieve a certain goal by cutting out all food. An anorexic's food intake typically drops from the normal 1200-1500 calories to 300-600 calories a day. With eating disorders, studies show that a healthy diet and exercise program is not enough to combat the disease; the person suffering from an eating disorder needs nurturing to have a void filled by something meaningful, something other than food.

Some eating disorder symptoms are 20 percent loss of body weight, loss of menstrual period, thinner hair, dry flaky skin, constipation (which will often be combated by excessive use of laxatives), lower blood pressure, lower potassium levels (the cause of singer Karen Carpenter's death), and a lower pulse rate. Dieting will become the most important thing in a person's life, and it may be coupled with excessive exercising. Most women who suffer from anorexia or bulimia will deny that there is anything wrong with their eating habits. Leading psychologists say that this disease could be overcome if the important people in the lives of anorexics and bulimics would let them know how valuable they are, regardless of their size. Victory over eating disorder syndromes is attainable, however. The success stories from women who have fought the battle and overcome this disease through the power of the Lord can be greatly encouraging.

Cherry Boone O'Neil loved being the daughter of Pat Boone but hated the pressure of being in the public eye.

That spotlight, coupled with her desire to be the "perfect daughter," nearly killed her. She was seventeen years old when her mother realized that Cherry's appearance was reminiscent of the photographs of Auschwitz inmates. She battled with anorexia and bulimia for ten years and, through the encouragement of her husband Dan and psychiatrist Dr. Ray Vath, Cherry was on the road to recovery. Today, she is fully cured; Cherry and Dan are the proud parents of five healthy children.

My friend Debbie has also battled with anorexia. She truly believed that she was "fat" although she naturally is one of the smallest framed people I know. When Debbie got married, she and her husband were told they probably would not have any children because of her experience with anorexia. Through the loving support of her husband, their close friends, church counselors, and the power of the Lord, Debbie overcame the disease. The Lord healed her completely, and now she and her husband Michael have been blessed with five beautiful children.

CONTENTMENT AND STRENGTH

Contentment comes when we exercise our wills to walk in obedience to the Lord. This involves more than soul searching; it involves knowing Him and "seeking His face." Then, "As you have therefore received Christ Jesus the Lord, so walk ye in Him." As our behavior patterns this, the fruit of the Holy Spirit is manifested in our lives: love, joy, peace, gentleness, goodness, faithfulness, teachability, patience, and self-control. As the husband and father demonstrates love to his wife in the same way that Christ loved the Church and gave himself for it, and the children obey their parents and act with respect and love toward one another, the home glorifies the Lord. When the home functions with the fruit of the Holy Spirit in operation, the family members influence their neighborhood to the glory of God. Through the family God will be glorified through to the community.

Modern America defines a successful mom as a "super-mom" who achieves everything from being CEO of her company to fashion designer, magazine editor, concert pianist, ballerina, and first-place winner in quilting at the county fair. A "successful dad" is one who pays the price to achieve "financial stability for his family." In most cases, the "supermom" and "successful dad" have sacrificed valuable family relationships for their "success." The Lord's idea of success is different from the world's idea of success. The Lord prefers obedience to sacrifice and measures success by obedience to His leading and direction.

The "seeming sacrifice" actually massages the egos of the "supermom" and the "successful dad" and amounts to partial obedience to God's Word instructing parents. Partial obedience carries the penalty of losing our influence over our children. Trying to live up to the "supermom" and "successful dad" models lead to the trap of monitoring success by comparison rather than God's standard for success. God places a higher standard upon the lives of those that He calls to be leaders. Scripture charges parents to rear their children in the "nurture and admonition of the Lord" and not to be a stumbling block them.

This past year I studied the life of Moses. I was most convicted by the incredibly high and separate standard the Lord places on those whom He calls to lead. Although we do not lead a whole nation, we are leading the next generation—our children—and we must raise them by example in the ways of the Lord. When Moses disobeyed God's command to speak to the rock by hitting the rock in anger (see Num. 20:8–13) and displaying disobedience to God before the people, God severely disciplined Moses by not allowing him to enter the promised land. Children can be trained through words, but they

are most highly influenced by example. When I am
ungodly before my children, I must fall to my knees
before the Lord and seek forgiveness from Him and also
from my children. The grace of our Lord Jesus Christ for-
gives my sins and empowers me to live a godly life before
my children. I'm not perfect, but my God is.

How vital it is that we obey the Lord rather than
deceive ourselves that we are "sacrificing for our families" and spend all our quality time away from them.
Sometimes you may wonder how to tell whether you are
walking in obedience or self-gratifying sacrifice. I realize
that if I walk in obedience to the Lord, then I experience
harmonious relationships within my family and within
my local church. When God's, peace reigns in my heart
over the difficult decisions that I must make every day,
then I keep short accounts with God, by confessing and
abandoning any sin which the Holy Spirit brings to my
attention. This keeps my focus on the Lord and guards
against the natural tendency to worship someone or
something more than I worship God.

Finding contentment and strength in the Lord leads
to freedom from the burden of comparison and dissatisfaction. Then the Lord will shine through our actions
and attitudes to the little eyes who watch and the little
ears who listen.

chapter seven

KIDS ARE
COPY CATS

This image of Jordan Ruth still makes me laugh. I walked into my bathroom one evening and there she was with my size 7 1/2 aerobic shoes on her feet, flossing her teeth, and doing crunches. She looked up and said, "Look, Mom, I'm exercising just like you." Now I see why Steve couldn't stop laughing when he saw my "routine" on our wedding night. (It is a funny sight, but *it works!*)

Johnston loves to put on "outfits" and entertain. Many of our guests have heard a "concert by Johnston," which is always *his* idea. One of my favorite performances was the night that Johnston donned Steve's cowboy boots and golf hat, packed a suitcase, created his own "airplane," and said, "I'm going to New York to do a concert! I'm there! Now I'm going to sing!" And he started singing!

Proverbs 17:6b says, "The glory of sons [or daughters] is their fathers [or mothers]!" The highest form of admiration is imitation. Our children watch our every move, and although we may be unaware of a habit or action, they seem to have memories like elephants! Steve and I have watched our children imitate our exercise and eating habits, our vocation, and our character qualities. Kids can't be fooled! If they don't see a character quality in us, then we won't see it developed in them.

I'm so thankful to my grandmother for encouraging me to read a chapter from the Book of Proverbs every day. Since there are thirty-one chapters in Proverbs, I read through the book twelve times a year. Reading Proverbs everyday has increased my determination to guard against the natural tendencies to get frustrated, to "lose control," and to be inconsistent with our children. I consider Proverbs my guardbook for God's wisdom in crucial times of crisis and in small, daily decisions.

My deepest desire is to make wise choices and to walk in integrity before my children. But how can I safeguard against my natural tendencies to get frustrated, lose control, and be inconsistent? Let's look more closely at the Book of Proverbs for the resources a parent requires for moral fitness.

CONSISTENT DISCIPLINE

"The rod and reproof give wisdom, but a child who gets his own way brings shame to his mother" (Prov. 29:15). Prayerfully seeking true wisdom will produce consistency, the bedrock of child discipline. Consistent discipline and definite boundaries communicate security and love to children. As we consistently follow through with what is best for their growth and development, our kids learn to trust us. Children may seem satisfied with "having their own way" at the time, but this pattern will produce a lack of trust in authority. That can eventually lead to immoral behavior—and shame to the family and a great burden to that child.

At the end of a very long day a comedy of errors erupted at our dinner table. I thought that everyone was eating well and conversing energetically when Jordan

Ruth decided it would be fun to make her chair fall over backwards. Maxfield and Johnston then got under the table and pretended that it was a spaceship—while Maxfield's placemat was pulled off the table in the process, spilling everything and Marshall threw his pudding and drink on the floor and Mary Morris started crying. All at once, all of the children except Mary Morris, needed correction. I was almost finished eating and *so* tired when my friend Cindy asked, "How do you do this?"

I looked around, smiled and said, "I just keep eating my dessert . . . !" We laughed! I had absolutely zero motivation to discipline with discretion. Instead, I felt like shouting orders. In the knick of time, however, the Lord reminded me of Proverbs 29:15, and I had the energy to discipline the children with consistency.

Parenting takes a lot more energy and self-discipline than anything that I have ever done before, but as it is with all things that are hard in the process, the results are well worth it! Every day I find myself singing as a constant reminder, "The joy of the Lord is my strength," and "Rejoice in the Lord always and again I say rejoice!" We need to find our joy (it's not the same as happiness) in Christ. Joy is the overflowing contentment that we find when we rest in the fact that God is in control. Then we, through Christ, can be faithful to do what we know is right out of a genuine love for our children instead of letting the moment pass by.

GODLY INSTRUCTION

"Train up a child in the way that He should go and when he is old, he will not depart from it" (Prov. 22:6). What a challenging promise for parents! A mother is not only a nurturer but also a provider of daily needs, including the child's need of instruction. What an awesome responsibility we have as parents!

Our Sunday school teacher shared a story of a small-town couple who went on vacation. Since they had not ventured far from their secure "Christian" town, the couple set ground rules before leaving on their trip. One was that they would boycott any restaurant that served alcohol. Stopping at a small diner, the husband kept the motor running while the wife ran in and popped the question. The man behind the counter replied, "No, ma'am, we're in a dry county, but we can buy a good beer from the private club next door if you'll stay and eat!" Well, she looked at him in shock and said, "No, thank you! With those standards, you don't deserve our business!"

This story is a clear example of how two people can hear the same question, interpret it two ways, and anticipate completely different answers. This is how it is with our children. We are called to train them in the *way* that *they* should go. Each child is unique. We may give the same verbal instruction to two children and each will interpret it differently—in his or her own way. As parents we must *know* our children and not try to conform them to our personalities; instead we must equip them to grow into the man or woman that God has uniquely designed! Godly character qualities "caught" by the child from the parent are meshed into that God-given destiny. Training by example far outweighs training by verbal command without godly example. Josh McDowell told Steve and me after Maxfield was born, "Rules without relationship lead to rebellion." We seek to establish a loving relationship with our children so that the boundaries we set are cushioned with grace and love.

SLOWNESS TO ANGER

"He who is slow to anger is better than the mighty, and he who rules his Spirit than he who captures a city" (Prov. 16:32). Responding to our children in anger is the quickest way to build disrespect. For our children to develop godly, moral behavior, they must have a healthy respect for authority and a thriving relationship within the family. The greatest laboratory for growing moral fiber is the home. Parents provide the environment where kids feel the freedom to "test the waters" and to ask questions within the boundaries set for each child. A hostile environment where any "wrong" move receives an angry parental response produces a stagnant, rigid home where children are so restrained that they will "test the waters" elsewhere and cause embarrassment to their parents. When I reach my limit as a mom, I remember this verse. The easy way out is to yell and control; the stronger, effective way is to stop, pray, and then deal with the situation for each child as God leads. When I allow myself to "fly out of control," the children get the upper hand; but when I respond in a calm and controlled manner, the children learn to take responsibility for their actions in future situations.

BUILDING RELATIONSHIPS

I was talking with a couple recently who have a twenty-one-year-old daughter who is not walking with the Lord. They are a wonderful Christian family, and their other two children are walking with the Lord. I was sharing with them several of the principles that Steve and I are trying to live out in our home. Yet with our oldest child being only six, I wondered what I would write twenty years from now when our children are grown.

I asked if they could give us some insight on parenting. They said that as they looked back the only difference that they saw in their parenting of their twenty-one-year-old daughter, who is the middle child, and their other children is that they did not spend as much focused time with her as the others (which of course they did not realize at the time). They also wish that they would have been more consistent with making sure their children got along with each other. As a parent of small children, this advice is a valuable nugget of wisdom.

"A fool does not delight in understanding, but only in revealing his own mind. . . . Before destruction the heart of man is haughty, but humility goes before honor. He who gives an answer before he hears it is folly and shame to him" (Prov. 18:2, 12–13). My friend Amy has the gift of focusing on her conversation partner, even in a crowded room full of friends. Amy has the quality of thoughtfulness and the ability to remember even the smallest of details that you share with her. She is more interested in understanding what you think and want to discuss, rather than in telling you her ideas and discussing subjects of her own interest. Through Amy's example, I have renewed my commitment to listen to what another person is trying to communicate—and another person includes my child. Getting eye level with the children when they are talking helps me to listen and not to be distracted. Otherwise, I find myself trying to listen while I continue doing several other things.

I have learned volumes about communication from my Grandaddy Carloss, who is a warm, walking encyclopedia of information. I could introduce him to a friend of mine, and Grandaddy would prompt them to share their interests and respond with several specific stories relating to those interests. He has so many accomplishments and interests that the conversation could easily center on him; but he has this quiet, godly way of answering the question and then naturally turning the conversation back to the other person. He has been a constant example of true humility.

If we can lay down our pride and walk humbly in our relationship with our spouse and with our children, then these relationships will naturally grow stronger. As we *listen*, we become sincerely interested in what the other has to say rather than in voicing our own opinion. We really hear not just the words, but the need behind the words; and we build trust in our relationships.

Our children are called first to obey, and then to honor their parents. Honoring parents is a command with a promise of long life. Proverbs tells us that *humility* comes *before* honor. If we desire to have kids that honor us as they grow into adolescence and adulthood, then we must first display genuine humility in our lives and relationships. Listening and walking in humility are the backbone of developing moral fitness.

LOVING OUR SPOUSE

"An excellent wife, who can find? For her worth is far above jewels. The heart of her husband trusts in her and he will have no lack of gain. She does him good and not evil all the days of her life" (Prov. 31:10–13). One of the greatest gifts a mother can give her children is to love their father. Through the marriage relationship, children learn what to look for in a mate. More than half of our children's lives will probably be spent in a marriage and parenting relationship. Studies have shown that the home environment has the greatest influence on a person's moral development. Our moral character determines what kind of mate we choose, and that choice is one of the three most important decisions that a person makes. The most important is accepting or rejecting Christ. The second is the choice of vocation, and the third is the choice of a marriage partner.

The relationship between the mom and the dad sets the tone for the household; a loving relationship provides stability in the home. Kids learn comraderie with one another from watching their parents, and they sense when it is missing. The greatest gift that we can give our children is a healthy, vibrant relationship with our spouse that is rooted in the Lord Jesus Christ.

Well, I could close the chapter here, but several of my friends have raised the question, "This all sounds really nice and easy, but what if I don't have a good relationship with my husband, or we don't really have a Christian home, or I'm a single parent?"

Without going into a lot of detail, Steve and I have been down some rocky roads. Thankfully because of God's grace and our commitment to marriage for a lifetime, the tough times were not devastating times. Instead the realization that things weren't as perfect and as wonderful as we'd dreamed they would be brought growth and depth to our marriage. Now we wouldn't trade the tough times for a million fairytales. Through talking to other couples and reading several books, we discovered that most marriages hit some real trying times at certain stages. The Lord has protected our marriage from outside affairs, although we have been faced with temptations. Anyone faced with temptation must do as Joseph did with Potiphar's wife (see Gen. 39) and *flee!* Changing partners only exchanges one set of problems for another.

No matter how impossible marriage may seem at times, God uses it to sharpen us and to conform us to the image of His Son. The rewards are great, as the Lord has brought our marriage to a deeper and more intimate level. God continues to weave us together. So don't give up! When you feel defeated and your friends advise you to take the kids and *leave*, seek the Lord. He will give you the strength and the wisdom to walk through the "impossible" into the incredible experience that He intended when He created marriage. (In the case of physical or sexual abuse, however, professional counseling must be sought. When abuse involves children, you must take action immediately.)

I had a wonderful Sunday school teacher in high school. Marge grew up in a home with a Christian mother and an alcoholic father. Marge came to the Lord at an early age. Although many would call her home dysfunctional, her mother sought the Lord's strength and heeded the verse in 1 Peter 3:1, 3–4, "In the same way, your wives, be submissive to your own husbands so that even if any of them are disobedient to the Word, they may be won without a word by the behavior of their wives. . . . And let not your adornment be merely external . . . but let it be the hidden person of the heart, with the imperishable quality of a gentle and quiet spirit, which is precious in the sight of God." After many years of faithfulness by Marge's mother, her father came to the Lord at the age of sixty-seven. He lived twenty more years, and Marge says that her mom vows that the joy of the last twenty years has far outweighed the first forty-five years of pain. So if you're in an unequally yoked marriage, then cling to the Lord for His strength to stay faithful in the midst of a frustrating and seemingly impossible situation. When you get discouraged, remember Marge's mom as tangible evidence that God really can turn hopeless situations into miracles!

My dad had many wonderful qualities, but he and my mom had a generally rocky marriage. Except for the early years, he was not a daily part of my life. He was there for special occasions and incredible family vacations, but basically my mom reared my sister and me as a single parent. The Lord faithfully provided in many ways. I saw the positive side of their relationship growing up, and although I was aware that there was conflict, I had a healthy view of marriage from watching them together. My mom stood on biblical principles in her relationship with my dad and never stopped praying and believing that God would do a miracle in their relationship. This was a living picture of commitment in marriage, no matter what!

Also, my grandparents were a stable part of our lives, and my grandfather gave me that consistent male influence and attention that growing girls so desperately need. My mom was faithful in prayer and reminded us through her words and actions that God is always a faithful Husband and Father especially when our earthly husband/father is not there. This powerfully impacted our lives, for she planted the seeds that our self-worth comes only from Christ. The Lord truly can "fill the gap" in your family if one parent is not there. Win this battle on your knees as you watch the Lord provide for the unfulfilled needs in your life and the lives of your children.

One final note on morality: Many "religions" emphasize the importance of being a good "moral" person. While we strive to raise morally fit kids and to display these qualities ourselves, we must beware that we do not allow morality to become our "god," that is, something that we take pride in becoming. This often happens when strong moral fiber is not grounded in spiritual truth. This is why the foundation of the totally fit life is not moral fitness, but first finding out what it means to be spiritually fit!

PART III

SPIRITUAL FITNESS

chapter eight

POWERFUL
RPMS

H eading off to college I heard a powerful statement, "Don't just learn how to make a living, but learn how to live a life!" I quickly learned that a life lived without a solid foundation was a shallow, lonely life. The summer before my freshman year in college I faced situations which tested my standards, and I learned to set boundaries that summer. I took classes to get a head start and tried to juggle the academic and social life of an eighteen-year-old with lots of opportunities and distractions. Just balancing my checkbook was quite a challenge!

I had allowed the urgent to overtake the important when I heard a speaker say that thirty minutes in the Word before studying was more valuable than hours in "the books." The most important part of my life, my walk with the Lord, had become secondary in light of the new demands on my daily schedule. Although I still read my Bible every day and prayed, I did it at the end of the day and would often fall asleep reading. Memorization of the Word had been replaced by memorizing for tests. This word of wisdom early in my college life, helped me set

75

my priorities straight before my new ways became a habit.

I had had a taste of motherhood prior to becoming a mom when I was a camp counselor—a twenty-four-hour parent to ten children. I learned to carry a little Bible around in my shorts and read whenever I had the chance. I wrote in my journal only twice that month, and I memorized only one verse. Through this experience, I learned to be more flexible in my walk with the Lord. I realized that He looks at the condition of our hearts and not just the outcome of our actions to determine where we are with Him. After camp, I went back to "normal life"— thankful for what I had learned and treasuring the experience—but I was glad to resume my regular schedule!

When Steve and I became parents for the first time, we realized that camp was now "normal life" and we would be parents for the rest of our lives. Although our new baby was a welcome member of our home who would "fit into and not control" the family, this precious little life would indeed change our lives forever! Now I needed to learn how to be a mom and still maintain a consistent walk with the Lord.

How does a mother do that? Read the Word, pray, and memorize Scripture! These are the three essentials to every vibrant walk with the Lord. Let's look at some practical ways to keep our spiritual motor maintained consistently in the ever-changing environment of motherhood.

READ!

Everytime I sit down for a few minutes I usually fall asleep, especially when I am reading. I convinced myself that I wouldn't be able to read again until Maxfield was old enough to read, because I was so tired when he was two weeks old. I could not stay awake to read the Bible, even though I knew that spending time alone in the

Word is the most powerful growth factor in my relationship with Jesus Christ.

I experienced an abrupt halt to my usual pattern of
reading through the Bible, which had included a chapter
from the Old Testament, a chapter from the New Testament, three to five Psalms (depending on how long they
were), and one Proverb every day. After a few weeks, I
finally began to read while I nursed; just as I had read a
proverb a day aloud to Maxfield when I was pregnant, I
did the same while nursing. Once he was sleeping
through the night I awakened early and spent time with
the Lord in the morning; and in the evening, I read a
chapter from my current favorite book and a devotional
before going to sleep.

This method worked for a while until we started having more children. By the time our third child joined our
family, I was definitely living on "yesterday's manna,"
which is a term often used by my friend Davita to
describe walking with the Lord and ministering to others
without spending time in the Word. "Yesterday's manna"
is available to those who have a lot of head knowledge of
the Bible, but just as the Israelites collected fresh manna
every morning to avoid eating food filled with maggots,
so we must be strengthened by a daily intake of God's
Word.

The Lord faithfully reminded me of advice that Ruth
Graham had given me years earlier after I told her that I
wanted several children. Ruth said that she kept an open
Bible in her kitchen and in her family room to read
whenever she had a moment. Ruth's respected husband,
Billy Graham, once was asked, "What would you do to
reach the world with the gospel, if you had only five years
to live?" He answered, "I would spend four years studying
and one year telling." The advice of the Grahams helped
me to keep my priorities straight in a practical way. I
have been able to take advantage of those moments of

opportunity to read a proverb to the kids or to teach them a new verse. I've found that the early afternoon is the best time for my personal study, which is possible during the children's quiet time. If I don't have the Bible open and accessible, the distractions of "life" will overtake my study time—and I will find myself reading at midnight and falling asleep with the light on and an open Bible in my lap.

PRAY

"Mom, I want to pray!". . . "No, Mom, it's my turn to pray!" . . . "Jordan Ruth always gets to pray!" This is a typical dialogue at the Camp house during meal time. Just six months ago we tried to encourage the children to pray out loud at the dinner table. Now, who gets to pray has surpassed who gets to ride in the front seat of the car! When our children see that prayer is a regular and real part of our lives, they will make it a consistent part of their lives as well.

When I was building friendships and starting to grow in the Lord, my grandaddy reminded me that I wouldn't get to know someone if I didn't spend time with them. So how can I know the Lord if I fail to spend time with Him in prayer? Granddaddy also added that a vital part of a growing relationship is listening. Not only do I need to start each day talking with the Lord, but I need to listen for His answers.

Well, all this sounds great unless you have children with a built-in alarm clock that says, "Mom's up!" It seems that whether I awaken at 5 A.M. or 7 A.M., someone decides to "wake up" with me. I even have literally tried going into my closet, but a few minutes later Jordan Ruth will appear looking for a pair of my shoes to play "dress up." My mother has been a real inspiration to me in this area because I remember many times walking into her room and finding her on her knees. Whenever I shared a problem or concern with her, we first went together to the Lord in prayer to seek His wisdom in the situation. I pray that as our kids get older they will see this same example in Steve and me.

But—while they are toddlers—I've sought lots of advice in this area and I've learned the true meaning of "praying without ceasing." Starting when I roll out of bed in the morning, continuing during those quiet moments in the shower (which are *most* productive), through that wonderful time when the kids are asleep in the car or during their quiet times, until I fall asleep at night—each day, I pray and see the Lord teaching and listening.

Have you ever said, "I'll pray for you" and then two weeks later you see the person and remember, "Oh! I meant to pray." This really started happening when I had kids because I've become convinced that a woman loses a part of her memory with each child—or maybe it's just that we have so much more to remember! After our first child was born, the Lord convicted me of praying right away when I promise to pray for someone or something; and then the Lord reminds me to pray throughout the day for certain individuals who need prayer.

After getting pregnant with our fourth child, I had a hard time spending concentrated time in prayer. The Lord used my dear friend Mary's example of faithfulness in prayer to encourage me to keep focused prayertime central in my life. It wasn't through Mary's direct comments on prayer, but through praying with her and seeing the evidence of focused prayertime with the Lord that challenged me to fervently seek that time in my own life. Now the Lord will often awaken me at 3 or 4 A.M. for prayer time (and I think that He was preparing me for the first few weeks of waking up with little Mary Morris!). That is a great opportunity for prayer because you're definitely too tired to read! That's when He gives me time to listen and hear His incredible answers. Afterwards, I can go back to sleep until morning "officially" arrives and it's amazing how refreshed I feel. Since this has started happening from time to time, I've met several other women who have said that very early morning is their best time to pray. They also found that the Lord would always give supernatural energy the next day or provide a time to take a long nap.

In this flexible season of life, the Lord's faithfulness continues to amaze me! It shouldn't, though, because He promises that He is always faithful—even when I am not (2 Tim. 2:13)—but I continue to marvel at His ways. When I start to become anxious He shows me things, such as making every traffic light green as I drive to church on Sunday morning and I am praying to be on time. Then I see that in the smallest of details, He is listening and faithfully answering my prayers!

MEMORIZE

There is a difference between memorizing and engrafting something into your heart. I am very good at learning something for a test or a speech and then one week later forgetting everything that I once knew so well. It seems that I'm not alone in this arena. Although people like my husband and my sister (who is blessed with my father's photographic memory) can read something once and remember it forever, for those of us not gifted in this area of memorizing, there are paths to victory! We must not use our lack of natural talent in this area as an excuse to avoid hiding God's Word in our hearts. To get motivated in this discipline, we must first examine how important it is to memorize Scripture.

"Thy Word is a lamp unto my feet and a light unto my path" (Ps. 119:105). As the well-loved psalm says, God's Word must guide our paths. It's hard to walk and read! So as we hide God's Word in our hearts, His Word guides *every* step of our lives. The Bibles can all be taken away, but no one can take the Word of God that has been engrafted in our hearts!

I asked Joe White—director of Kanakuk Kamps and a gifted author, speaker, and very wise and respected father of four teenage and young adult kids—"What is the key to raising kids that turn out like yours?" He said, "Without a doubt, it's teaching them God's Word at a very early age."

We began to teach Maxfield Psalm 23 when he was three. Johnston and Jordan Ruth began learning Bible verses at two years of age. I'd like to say that we learn a verse a week and give you an easy formula to follow, but I have found that sometimes it takes a month to *really* learn just *one* verse; and other times a verse "clicks" the first week and is hidden in the heart forever. If we're learning a chapter like Psalm 23, we might take an occasional break from it and memorize something applicable and easy like, "I will obey God's Word" (Ps. 119:17b), which is Maxfield's favorite verse. One practical way to learn a verse is to write it on a three-by-five card and carry it with you. It's great to have it in the car when you're driving carpool and review it with your kids and their friends (the carpool Bible).

Memorization is definitely the weakest area in my life. Whether it is learning God's Word or remembering names, I find it a constant challenge; but I'm thankful that the Lord promises that where I am "weak," He is "strong." He has taught me so much about leaning on Him and about the importance of accountability not just in the easy areas, but in those places where I am weak. "For as we hide God's Word in our hearts, it protects us from falling into sin and as we obey His commands, He cleanses our way" (Ps. 119:9,11, TLB).

I've been thankful for advice on how to balance these areas with motherhood, but I've had an underlying concern that these seasonal habits will become lifelong. I was so encouraged by my friend Mel who has kids seven and nine. She shared that the Lord had just recently convicted her that the "spiritual maintenance while having small children" season of her life was over and now she needed to spend more devoted and focused time with the Lord each day. We must remember that our children are small for only a short while. The Lord will show us when we can resume a more focused time in the Word, prayer, and memorization.

THE SERVANT LEADER

The three wise men expected to find a baby born to be King of the Jews. How amazed they must have been to find a young child who was born in a stable instead of a palace, where He was surrounded by shepherds instead of soldiers, and welcomed by a carpenter and his wife kneeling by a feeding trough instead of a king and queen kneeling by a cradle made of gold.

Here was the child who would change the course of history—entering our world in a way so unassuming, yet noticed not by those heralded by kings but by those called of God. Jesus, born to die, served His parents for thirty years before He embarked on His ministry to serve many. He lay down His life on a cross at the hill called Golgotha and then was victoriously resurrected and lives in the lives of those whom He would save for eternity.

The greatest leaders are focused on serving the needs of others rather than leading people in their own direction. Jesus is our greatest example; as He served and gave Himself to others, He forever changed lives lived before, during, and after His short time on earth. It is naturally easier for us to be served than to serve. Well, let me restate that—it is naturally easier for us to be served than to genuinely serve without having our own agenda. This freedom to give ourselves to others becomes a part of our character as we grow in Christ.

Motherhood is definitely a lesson in servanthood. Babies are completely dependent for survival on the care of another, and they need loving stimulation to grow into healthy, balanced children. Even when children learn patience, sharing, and the importance of looking out for others besides themselves, they still need our confirming love, time, and attention. The family is the initial framework in which we grow and learn how to relate to others, and the family is where the last three vital areas of spiritual growth begin.

First, we need each other. The call in Hebrews 10:24–25 is to *fellowship:* "consider how to stimulate each other to love and good deeds, not forsaking our assembling together, as is the habit of some, but encouraging one another, and all the more, as you see the day drawing near." Then, we must reach out to others through *evangelism* and *discipleship!* In Matthew 28:19–20 we find the familiar Great Commission, "Go ye therefore and make disciples of all nations, baptizing them in the name of the Father, Son and the Holy Spirit, teaching them to observe all that I commanded you, and lo, I am with you always, even to the end of the age." Let's see why and how these areas are part of the spiritually fit foundation that will lead to success in the physical and moral fitness areas of life.

FELLOWSHIP

Spending time with other Christians allows us to reach our greatest potential. Growth happens through being a part of a specific church body. I have a friend who had a bad experience with the "organized church" growing up. In college, she developed a personal relationship with Jesus Christ, but she had a hard time feeling comfortable in an actual church and felt that she could grow in the Lord on her own. She justified her refusal to join a church by dwelling on her childhood experience. When she married and started a family, she and her husband realized how vital it was to attend a church. They found a strong Bible-based church and now she can clearly see what she had been missing all these years. The church provides stability and general accountability for them, not only through the pastor and leaders in the church, but also through other families who walk down similar paths and can relate to their victories and struggles in life.

The church setting provides opportunity for deeper relationships to grow. There is a difference in fellowshipping with a group of people and being in a discipleship relationship. Fellowship is community sharing in an interest or activity which may result in discipleship. Part of discipleship is teaching another how to initiate fellowship. How does this look practically, and how can it relate to "total fitness"?

Check out these ideas! A group of women combine prayer and Bible study with doing a video workout tape (like the *Lifersize* workout!). Also, any outdoor activity such as long walks or park picnics, snow skiing, or a summer beach trip are great opportunities to know other families and to experience life situations that aren't discoverable in a sit-down Bible study.

Fellowship within the family unit builds a vital foundation for deeper relationships within the family. As we will spend time doing fun things together, we realize that these times are productive and significant. Some nights we feel as if we're just "getting through dinner" with everyone needing a drink refill at different times and asking questions like, "How much more do I have to eat before I can have dessert?" So, instead of dreading mealtime, we plan fun things by having picnics and cookouts outside and carpet picnics if it is raining. Occasionally, we have "formal" dinner parties with roses and candle-light and "extra special manners" in the dining room. Children learn more by living life with us than by listen-ing to our words of wisdom.

Times of fellowship are also great times to invite non-Christian or unchurched friends to come and be exposed to some good, clean fun! This leads to our next area, *evangelism*.

EVANGELISM

A multitude of information is available on leading oth-ers to Christ! When we first come to the Lord, we learn the salvation verses such as John 3:16, Romans 3:23 and 6:23, and 1 John 1:9 (to name a few). Then we're ready to tell others about our newfound faith.

My husband Steve has the gift of making one think on a deeper level about something that they have assumed or believed. Steve often compares evangelism to an engagement. When you meet the one you want to marry, you are so deeply in love that most people have to tell you to *stop* talking about that person, not teach you what to say! This is how we should be in our relationship with the Lord. When our life is built on the foundation of a healthy, growing relationship with Christ, then people will see the evidence in our lives.

My friend Mary and I cochaired a charitable fundrais-ing event last year and worked with an incredible team of women from different walks in life. After the event, one woman commented that there was obviously something different about the way that we handled stressful situa-tions. She knew that we were both Christians and asked if that was what made a difference in the way that we handled stress—and if she and her husband could visit our church with us. Mary and I were not consciously trying to act a certain way, but the Lord living through us made an impact.

This year our church decided to move Vacation Bible School (VBS) from the church to the homes of the members. Backyard Bible Clubs were held in different neighborhoods around the city. My friend Joan opened her home and many of her friends brought their children who probably would not have brought them to the church for VBS. The last day, Johnston brought home a bracelet that he made with different color beads. The *black* was for sin; the *red* bead signified Jesus' blood covering our sin; the *white* bead represented purity and righteousness before the Lord because of Christ's blood covering our sin; the *green* stands for growth which comes as we walk with Christ; and the *yellow* bead reminds us of God's promise of heaven. He loves to wear the bracelet, and it has become a wonderful tool for Johnston to share the gospel with his family and friends.

The home is where evangelism begins. I always thought that evangelism was going out and sharing Christ; however as a mom with five small children, I've found that my greatest mission field is right here at home. Our kids need to see Christ in us if we want them to come to know the Lord. I've found that it's easier to be godly outside the home, sharing Christ with non-Christians, and seeing them come to Christ. The real test, though, is living out the fruit of the Spirit at home. We want our children and their friends to see us growing in the Lord and to desire that growth for themselves.

DISCIPLESHIP

The Lord did not call us to "go into all the world and make converts" but to "go into all the world and make *disciples!*" When we have the privilege of being God's vehicle through the Holy Spirit to lead someone to the Lord, we are then responsible to follow up with discipleship. This does not mean that we must personally disciple all those whom we lead to the Lord, but we should "hook them up" with someone or a small group that will be faithful and consistent in their lives. The Lord has given women a model for discipleship in Titus 2:3–5, "Older women likewise are to be reverent in their behavior, not malicious gossips, nor enslaved to much wine, teaching what is good, that they may encourage young women to love their husbands, to love their children, to be sensible, pure, workers at home, kind, being subject to their own husbands, that the word of God may not be dishonored." We are each an older woman to someone, and there is always some one "older" than we are. If a younger woman is older spiritually and through experience, she could disciple someone older in actual age.

The Lord has faithfully provided the perfect person to disciple me at each stage in my life. Now that I'm a mom, I'm in a young mother's group with three other women, and we are discipled by a godly woman who has children in their teens and early twenties. Stephanie has the gift of seeing right where we are in life and when we are hurting. She is faithful to pray and hold us accountable to our spiritual goals. I had discipled junior high and high school girls until our fourth child Marshall was born. The Lord showed me that this was a season where I needed to focus on the ultimate discipleship—our own children! After all, I have a small group right here at home! Just as the goal for discipleship is to encourage women not to become dependent on us, but (as my husband Steve says) to be "co-dependent" on Christ, parents can equip children to live healthy, godly lives when they become adults.

CONCLUSION:
PERSPECTIVE PLUS

I t was 4 P.M. Friday afternoon, Labor Day weekend. My mom had just left to go to Austin to
meet my sister, and I was driving up to Lake
McQueeney with a friend the next day to meet them. My
adrenalin was going because I had lots of reasons to be
excited about the weekend. First, because I was "home
alone" and almost everyone in my extended family was
out of town, I had invited a lot of my friends over for a
party. Then, my family and I were going skiing all weekend and this fun guy that I had a crush on was going with
us. Most of all, I was anxious to get back from skiing
because I had listened to my parents' conversation the
night before (after they thought that I had hung up the
phone) and Dad and Mom had decided that on Tuesday,
September 8, he would move back to Houston and they
would get back together. In the midst of this excitement,
the phone rang. It was my dad.

"Kim, have a great time skiing this weekend. I'll see
you on Tuesday. I'm heading to Fort Lauderdale, Florida,

to meet the president for an economic conference we're doing together. (Dad was President Reagan's executive economic advisor at that time.) Wish you were going with me, but I know you'll have fun at the lake. Oh, hang on. I have to run. Priscilla is on the other line needing to work out some details for the promo tour next month. (Priscilla Presley. Dad had been good friends with Elvis, and he was trustee for Lisa Marie's estate and an advisor to Priscilla after Elvis's death. They had just opened Graceland to the public, and he and Priscilla were preparing for a promotional tour to the Orient in October.) We'll talk more next week. I love you! Remember to call Dearie (my grandmother, his mom) today. It's her birthday! Bye, love you too!"

I'm sure that I said something, but all I remember are his words. I don't remember them because of the important people he was interacting with—those were everyday events for Dad. I will forever remember his words because that was our last conversation and it was so quick and superficial. How I wish that I had known. I wonder what I would have said or what I would have asked. Instead, we just hung up the phone, and I quickly went back to preparing for the weekend. What more was there to say? I would see him on Tuesday.

The phone rang at 6 P.M. It was my grandfather, Dr. J.R. He said that I should sit down, and I asked if my grandmother was okay. He answered, "Yes, but sit down." Then he uttered piercing words, "Your father's plane has crashed and there are no survivors." Numbly, I hung up the phone to call the small Kansas City private airport. I insisted on talking to someone who had seen him get on the plane—to make sure that it was really my dad flying the plane.

I remembered the time during the hot summer of 1979 when Mom, Dad, Meredith, and I were flying home from camp with our heavy trunks in the cargo compartment—and an engine went out. Mother started praying for cool air to increase our air speed so that we could safely land at the Kansas City airport; the indicator showed an increase in air speed. We landed, and the other engine shut off immediately on touchdown; we had to be towed to the hanger. From time to time Dad had incidents like this and even worse, but he always safely landed the plane. What could have happened this time?

I called a good friend and asked her to turn on the TV. She confirmed that news flashes had reported that Morgan Maxfield's plane crashed about 4:30 P.M. No survivors. Apparently, something had caused the engines to stop. He was heading for a field and then turned the plane to miss some children when the left wing hit a tree and the plane nose-dived into the ground and blew up. A lady on television was quoted as saying "Morgan Maxfield crashed his plane to save my children!"

It was true. I ran all over the house and gathered everything that Dad had ever given me and put it in a pile in my room and laid on top of it and cried. "Why? Why my Dad?" Then I saw my Bible on my desk and remembered a verse that I had quoted so freely to my friends when they were hurting, Romans 8:28, "And we know that all things work together for good to those who love God and are called according to His purpose." I realized that I had a choice to make. I could fall apart—I'm sure everyone would understand—or I could trust that Romans 8:28 is true and live it out for the first time in my own life. I went downstairs and sat at the piano to sing, "Give them all, give them all, give them all to Jesus, shattered dreams, wounded hearts and broken toys. Give them all, give them all to Jesus and He will turn your sorrows into joy!"

This was just the beginning of learning what it means to truly step out in faith and trust completely in the sovereignty of God. One of the most valuable lessons that I had learned from my mom was to go to the Lord in a crisis first before going to someone else. On September 4, 1981, I lived it out! I realized that I cannot build my life on people or things. I had said many times that I could make it through anything as long as I had my dad, but now I know that I can make it through anything as long as I have the Lord. He alone is the one lasting stability in my life. I don't know what will happen in the next fifteen minutes, but the Lord sees the big picture for all of eternity and promises to guide our every step.

At age seventeen, I was trying to figure out who I really was and what I really believed was important in life. I was faithful with the habits that were established early in life because I had been taught that these ways were essential. Although my family thought that I was doing great, inside I was falling apart. It's real easy to put on the right "show," but when a crisis hits, what's really inside is tested.

I can hardly count how many times that I have thanked the Lord for staying close by me when my heart had wandered so far away. I learned that acting on what you know is right even when your heart is not there is the right step. Even though it seems hypocritical, God promises that His Word will not return empty without accomplishing what He desires (see Isa. 55:11). When I was faced with tragedy, I called to the Lord and depended on His strength. Considering the worldly focus of my heart the year before Dad was killed, I should not have responded in that way. However, God's Word had taken root in my heart so that I did not become bitter against God. The indwelling of the Holy Spirit gives us the power to act on the Word of God by faith.

The rewards are great when you have a godly perspective. At Dad's funeral, Meredith and I were able to speak and sing, as well as attend the three other funerals of those that were killed in the crash. To get to those funerals we had to get in a small plane just like Dad's, so that was a good step of faith. Many people came to know the Lord through Dad's funeral and at his burial. Since Dad was a public figure, I was invited by many different groups to share what the Lord had done in my life. I continue to share what the Lord has taught me in hopes that others will prepare themselves through the power of God's Word to deal with life's unexpected events—even tragedies.

I know you've been wondering what all this has to do with healthy exercise and eating habits. The same principle for keeping spiritually fit also is true for staying physically fit. There are seasons when we don't feel like eating right and exercising and can justify those reasons easily. However, when we continue with healthy habits, our bodies stay toned and able to face physical challenges, especially unexpected ones.

We have already examined many of the rewards of staying physically fit—especially the reward of a healthy outlook on life and appreciation for how the Lord created our bodies. A good friend recently told me she is disgusted with her physical appearance; she hasn't liked any photographs of herself taken during the last six months. The way she feels about how she looks has affected all of her relationships and she says that she's an emotional wreck. She wondered whether the *Lifersize* program could help her. I said that for it to reap permanent results, she must first build a solid spiritual foundation. A consistent, focused walk with the Lord will build into her life the strength and discipline she needs to act on what she knows is right and the willpower to be consistent with healthy eating and exercise habits.

Being a mom is a lifetime commitment. Steve and I wanted to have a lot of children; actually, he wanted three kids and I wanted seven. So when we had our fourth child, Marshall, we decided not to have any more children after the problems that I had experienced—from constant sickness to a tear in my placenta and surgery. I started to get excited about rearing our children, and the Lord gave me the idea to share these *Lifersize* principles with ten- to eighteen-year-old girls, so I began putting that project together. For the first time I had peace about not having any more children. Marshall had just turned one and I was going through all the baby clothes, saving some for my sister Meredith and giving others away.

One Friday I suddenly realized that the date had passed for my regular menstrual cycle. In fact, I knew that I was very late. Steve was out of town and all the kids were asleep so I took a pregnancy test which was left over from the previous pregnancy one year before. There it was as plain as day—I was pregnant!

For the first time since Dad's death I cried out to the Lord, "Why, me? Why not Sara or Jane?" They *so* wanted to have a child! I wondered, "Our birth control had worked for twelve months. Why not last month?" I knew the Lord wanted to teach me something *big* because I couldn't imagine that this could be part of His ordinary plan. I remembered my friend who became pregnant with number six, when I found out that I was pregnant with number three (Jordan Ruth) and Johnston was just three months old. She didn't tell me for a month, because she said that she had to wait until she was excited. I had been on cloud nine with number three and had told "the world." *A baby is such a precious gift,* I had thought at the time. *How could she not be thrilled?* I was the one having kids twelve months apart, and *her* youngest was four. Well, now I understood why she waited a month to tell me.

So I stopped. Once again, I was home alone (well, without another adult!). The Lord was with me as I saw the big picture, and I tried to understand. Knowing the right response, but struggling to get my heart and emotions to line up with the knowledge in my head, I told myself, *There is a little life growing inside and God's timing is always perfect!* Again I must act on what I knew to be right even though my real emotions said no! Steve could not be reached for several hours, and I wanted to be excited when I told him the news. So I prayed, read the Word, and went to sleep.

Each time I found myself pregnant, I have always told Steve in a unique, fun way, and now each of the children have a creative story to tell. I wanted this fifth child to have a special story; so I sent Steve a fax from his number five child saying, "Dad, I can't wait to meet you in June! Call Mom!" Steve was in shock, of course, but he was so excited. He'd cancelled his appointment to "Dr. Chop" four times that year, and now he was thrilled! I shared with him my reactions and said that the Lord was working in my heart—but he had eight months and "counting" to get to the doctor. (We're still counting!)

Several months later, I told my friend Jane what the Lord had been teaching me. She and her husband have been trying to have a baby for a long time, and she has been through a lot of infertility surgery and testing, all without becoming pregnant. I was hesitant to share my feelings in much detail because I was sure that it would be hard for her to hear and understand. Although Jane longs to have a baby, she is such a godly, mature woman that her response to my story was simply to say, "The infertility struggle has taught me to trust in God's timing while maintaining a godly perspective on life." It was amazing that through opposite circumstances the Lord taught us the same truth. For we can make our plans, but God directs our steps (see Prov. 16:9).

I am now holding our precious baby girl! Mary Morris Camp was born on June 4, 1995. I love her *so* much and thank the Lord for her every day. I had a great pregnancy and delivery; Steve and I are ecstatic about being parents again of a newborn. After each baby our relationship grows deeper and more intimate. The kids all line up to hold her. They *love* her, and there is not even a hint of jealousy. (Thank You, Lord!) Our biggest problem—if you can call it a problem—is that our second son Johnston wants to stay home all the time so that he can hold the baby.

Being pregnant with Mary Morris motivated me to prepare and to film the pregnancy and recovery videos and to write this book—which would have been an adventure lost if I had not become pregnant. I was only planning to do a video/devotional with these *Lifersize* principles for teenage girls. Wow! We have an incredible God. His plan for our lives far outshines our own if we will submit to Him and allow Him to go before us and guide our every step!

Having a healthy, godly perspective on life gives us the desire to do what is best for our spirit, soul, and body. It gives us the strength to persevere and the motivation to be a living example to our kids. *Lifersize* enables us to model how to live life to our fullest potential!

In closing, I share this poem my mother-in-law Ruth had in an old Bible.

REFLECTION

I sat by her bed, we had prayed, we had read, and we talked of our Savior's great love.

How He came from the sky, came to suffer and die, and someday would take us above.

We see Jesus each day! Then, she'd venture to say, "And He sees us now, doesn't He, Mother?"

We see Him, blessed thought, but our eyes see Him not in the way that we see one another.

"But I see Him!" said she, "Just as plain as can be!" Well, then, how does He look, tell me true?!

She was silent and then, as she smiled once again, "Mother, I think He looks just like you!"

Oh, what prayer fills my heart and I felt the tears start, as I thought how weakly I live.

How impatient I get. How I worry and fret. And I prayed, "Blessed Father, forgive."

Fill my life with Thy power, everyday, every hour, that the eyes of this child watching me,

As I live, as I pray, by Thy Spirit each day, may indeed catch a vision of Thee!